11/02

carol guber's type2

Diabetes Life Plan

Broadway Books
New York

carol guber's type 2

Diabetes Life Plan

Take Charge, Take Care, and Feel Better than Ever

Carol Guber

with Betsy Thorpe

This book is not intended to take the place of medical advice from a trained medical professional. Readers are advised to consult a physician or other qualified health professional regarding treatment of their medical problems. Neither the publisher nor the author takes any responsibility for any possible consequences from any treatment, action, or application of medicine, herb or preparation to any person reading or following the information in this book.

Broadway Books titles may be purchased for business or promotional use or for special sales. For information, please write to: Special Markets Department, Random House, Inc., 1540 Broadway, New York, NY 10036.

BROADWAY BOOKS and its logo, a letter B bisected on the diagonal, are trademarks of Broadway Books, a division of Random House, Inc.

Visit our website at www.broadwaybooks.com

PRINTED IN THE UNITED STATES OF AMERICA

Library of Congress Cataloging-in-Publication Data

Guber, Carol.
[Type 2 diabetes life plan]
Carol Guber's type 2 diabetes life plan : take charge, take care
and feel better than ever / Carol Guber with Betsy Thorpe.— 1st ed.
p.   cm.
Includes bibliographical references and index.
1. Non-insulin-dependent diabetes—Popular works. I. Thorpe, Betsy. II. Title.

RC662.18 .G83 2002
616.4'62—dc21   2001043406

FIRST EDITION

Designed by Nicola Ferguson

ISBN 0-7679-0525-3

10   9   8   7   6   5   4   3   2   1

To my loving mother,
Edna S. Tuttleman

Contents

Acknowledgments

The diagnosis of diabetes has been accompanied by a mixed bag of blessings for me. The most notable is the opportunity to write this book. In doing so I have had the support, advice, and inspiration from many people both professionally and personally. I would not have this chance were it not for the very early encouragement of my agent, Angela Miller, and Harriet Bell. They had a vision of the diamond in the rough, which Angela has continued to develop.

Special thanks to the folks at Broadway Books: Trish Medved, my editor, Catherine Pollack, Brian Jones, James Benson, Liz DeRidder, and Nicola Ferguson.

Many nutrition and health professionals have contributed their expertise, information, and advice, including Gerald Bernstein, M.D., past president of the American Diabetes Association; Robin Goland, M.D.; Lisa Young, Ph.D.; Marie Scioscia, M.S., R.D.; Gayle Reichler, M.S., R.D.; Dana Sapio, M.S., R.D.; Lewis Mehl-Madrona, M.D., Ph.D.; Marion Franz, R.D., C.D.E.; Anne Daley, M.S., R.D., C.D.E.; Janelle White, M.D.; and Marion Nestle, Ph.D., M.P.H., department chair; and the faculty of the department of Nutrition and Food Studies, New York University.

Amber Devlin, Jeanne Ashby, and David Schab provided invaluable information.

I wish to acknowledge the help of the American Diabetes Association staff: Angela Russo, Bernadette King, Marie Kaplowitz, and Terence Knox.

Gratitude toward Roger Weiss, M.D., Michael Knowles, Ben

acknowledgments

Bailey, Joseph Martin, Shiraz Lebya, Sallie Ellis, William Scott, and Kyle Shadix.

Betsy Thorpe has demonstrated perseverance, humor, and a keen ability to understand the essence of an issue. Many thanks to her. And Betsy would like to thank her husband, Chris, for his love and support during the writing of this book, and her baby, Georgia, who would play patiently and nap well as her mommy typed and e-mailed.

I have been blessed with joyful friends and a rambunctious, loving family. Some friends have paved the way with books of their own: Mimi Sheraton, Sylvia Weinstock, Rozanne Gold, Lorna Sass, Dana Jacobi, Michelle Scicolone, Cara da Silva, and Irene Sax.

No one could ask for dearer friends in life than Margo Schab and Laura Keeler. Margo Feiden keeps watch 24 hours a day and Fern Berman believed in me before I knew why. Barbara Walters taught me how to have great friendships with women and loyalty where it counts.

To Stan Tuttleman, whose parenting has given me the foundation to go forth into the world. His commitment has afforded me the chance to fulfill my dreams. My sister Jan Tuttleman is a true friend and co-conspirator of wonderful adventures. Much love to my siblings: Zev and Heidi, Steven and Beth, David and Claudia and Jackie. Thanks to all my nieces and nephews: Marisa, Liz, Sarah, Sophie, Emma, Willa, Max, Sam, Justin, and Adam.

Finally to my son, Noah Shachtman, there is no one finer than you.

Introduction

Real life never seems to turn out the way we had imagined or planned. Love, marriage, career, children . . . it's likely that all of these have brought you highs and lows that you never anticipated. And whether your health has been excellent or poor until now, it is likely that you didn't expect a diagnosis of this chronic disease—diabetes. I was surprised to have developed diabetes, despite having a long history of it in my family: my mother has it, as did both my grandfather and great-grandmother. My great-uncle Shaya was an amputee because of it.

Whether or not your diabetes diagnosis came as a complete surprise, you might have known it was lurking in your family background, or you have been told you are "borderline." You may be wondering what to do *now*. I recommend a life plan, which is the basis of this book: Real life—in this case, diabetes—provides real possibilities. The first step to take is to acknowledge that life is messy and inspirational all at the same time, and therein lies the opportunity. This book encourages you to see diabetes as a chance to assess your life and change it for the better, to take charge and take care. The very nature of living well with diabetes encourages you to look anew at the most elemental activities in life: eating, exercising, communicating, and looking after yourself. In living well from this day forward with diabetes, you can make vital alterations in your mind, body, and spirit.

My Story

I was diagnosed with diabetes in September 1998. Although I was aware of my family's history of developing this disease, I thought I had a special shield against illness because I have a master's degree in nutrition and taught for many years in the Department of Nutrition and Food Studies at New York University. There was no way it could happen to me, as I studied and taught the effects of diet on health. With this knowledge, I thought I could keep all diseases at an arm's length. Well, knowledge may be power, but it wasn't enough to keep diabetes at bay. Four generations of genetics was stronger than my sense of denial.

I wasn't aware of any symptoms when I was diagnosed—it was discovered during a routine checkup. When my doctor called me with the news, I wasn't surprised and I wasn't devastated, at least at first. In fact, I felt very feisty and thought that I could take this disease head-on. It wasn't until days later that it began to dawn on me that this was a battle I was going to have to wage *forever*; that I might be able to control my illness but it was not going to go away. My doctor suggested taking medication to control the disease, but I wanted to wait and see if I could manage this by changing old lifestyle habits, which had likely affected my health in the first place (along with those family genes). I was able to quickly swing into action with the knowledge I had developed over my years of involvement with nutrition. I did not have to wait for an explanation of carbohydrates, proteins, and fats to understand the adjustments that were required to my diet. I was also fortunate to have the support and advice of many colleagues who have done research in food, obesity, and physiology.

By making lifestyle changes in diet and exercise, enlisting the support of friends, family, and coworkers, and re-igniting my own inner resources and determination, I took charge of the areas that diabetes responds positively to. And at the same time, I altered my point of view about my life. On the most basic level I realized that modifying my lifestyle was not about lowering my dress size, not about making cosmetic changes; this was about the very quality of the rest of my life, a stirring, fundamental shift of the mind, body, and spirit. I wanted to hold life in a more dynamic fashion that would allow greater possibilities despite and because of diabetes.

Why did I write this book? Well, you may have heard about a person who was diagnosed with a disease and how it changed her life. For some, the circumstances are so devastating that it clouds all subsequent events and that cloud is never lifted. Yet others use the disease as a wake-up call to alter their lives for the better. I hope to inspire you to use your diagnosis in that positive way. I have changed tremendously since I was first diagnosed three years ago. Looking inward, I made some life-altering decisions and moved outward from there. Now I have lost almost 37 pounds and kept it off. I also have developed a weekly exercise routine that includes boxing—yes, real boxing!

These changes have affected my life in a dramatic fashion. I was able to lose weight by formulating a program for myself—the one that I share with you in this book. Now, activities that once seemed to take enormous amounts of the limited energy I had, have now become a joyful routine. I always imagined I would have a more sedentary existence at this stage in my life. That has changed; I no longer think about sitting on the front porch and being inactive in my "golden years." I enjoy physical activity every day and look forward to learning new and fun ways of keeping fit. I'm even thinking of skiing next winter, which I had stopped doing after I split my ski pants on the slopes when I was 21!

Through the challenge of dealing with my own diabetes and doing research for this book, I realized that you can't manage an illness without paying attention to the entire person inside and out. Diabetes requires more than testing blood sugar or controlling food intake, which is why I have become increasingly interested in a more integrative approach to my health. This now includes stress management, connecting with nature in meditation, and discovering healing traditions such as yoga and massage. All have helped me to live well, and thus help me with my diabetes.

In my interactions with this disease, my self-esteem has risen. The confidence that I feel in living well with diabetes extends to other areas in my life, and it feels as if new avenues are opening up to me all the time. In this book, I take the clinical information that I have studied and turned it into something practical—paying attention to the nitty-gritty daily needs that people have. I know there is a huge chasm between just reading about something and actually applying it to the complicated world we live in, where people must balance so many aspects of life at the same time.

It's my goal to make you feel that there are others out there, having similar experiences. That is why I include my own story, my mother's, and those of people I have interacted with.

How to Use This Book

In *Carol Guber's Type 2 Diabetes Life Plan* you have a practical resource of useful information about type 2 diabetes coupled with inspiration that you can live life in a whole new, constructive manner by making changes in diet and exercise, exhibiting a passion for the moment, and deciding to have many adventurous experiences. Let yourself have this of life. Use your living with diabetes as a chance to make some inroads in areas that you are unsatisfied with or maybe just have never considered. Let's face it, either you make the shift toward a healthier you now or, down the road, the severe medical complications you can develop in ignoring your diabetes will force you to alter your life. In making the healthy changes suggested in this book now, you can have the experience of feeling powerful in your fight against diabetes.

The information for this book comes from several sources: nutritional information that I have taught in my classes, experiences from the support groups I have run for NYU's faculty and staff with type 2 diabetes, stories from individuals I have counseled, and, of course, my own experiences and those of my mother. In addition, I have consulted and interviewed prominent authorities on diabetes. Their input, as well as input from other experts in nutrition, health, and exercise physiology, has been invaluable. Staff at the American Diabetes Association, as well as their volumes of material, have been a great resource. I have developed this book to be straightforward in manner. Here you will not read a distant clinical observation. This book was developed out of living with diabetes. I know what it feels like to worry about your blood sugar, obsess about weight, and wonder where the energy will come from to go to the gym.

During my yearly checkup, my primary care physician, a truly caring individual, was bemoaning the lack of time he has to spend with each patient. The economics of health maintenance organizations have swept away the time required to get all the care we need from our doctors. From where can we get the information? This book is set up to give you much information and direct you to other sources where you can develop strategies for yourself.

Joanne came to see me for counseling. She had recently been diagnosed and was panicked. Other family members had diabetes and she was frightened of complications. Equally upsetting was her doctor's demand that she lose 30 pounds. Joanne had every reason not to do it. The New York Knicks should have hired her, because she had the best defense I have ever witnessed. Every suggestion was blocked with excuses that she needed to do things for other people and couldn't take time for herself. Finally, after allowing her to try every move possible, I asked her, "When is it going to be your time?"

Like so many of us, we have learned to put ourselves as a low priority. Sometimes it takes a diagnosis to have us stop and question the way we've structured our surroundings. Joanne started by enlisting the support of her family. She found that instead of driving her children to all their activities on Saturday, she could go to the gym and they could go with their friends in a car pool. This was the family's way of rallying for her. Three months and 10 pounds lighter, Joanne was feeling very sassy and the whole family survived the change in their routine quite nicely.

Now she has reached her 30-pound goal. Through the process of looking inside herself and making some changes in her priorities she developed a new rich, inner confidence that is reflected in her face.

It is my goal to have others feel so inspired, because I have seen firsthand what kind of devastating damage can result from diabetes. My mother was diagnosed with the disease 20 years ago. Today, at 80, her eyesight is greatly impaired because of the complications from diabetes, and she recently suffered a heart attack. I want to stay vigilant and not let that happen to others or to me. To that end I have written this book to be used as a companion to your interactions with your physician and diabetes educator.

Part 1 provides information on type 2 diabetes, including the nature of the disease and the complications that can result. The section concludes with information on how diabetes affects different populations: different ethnicities, genders, and ages. Consider this part of the book as a place where you can learn more about the disease and how it affects your body. Without possessing the knowledge of how this disease operates, it will be difficult for you to function well with diabetes. If you are a person who needs the background and facts before you start on anything, this is where you should start.

If you are anxious to begin changing your life for the better today, go to part 2, which covers practical ways to live with diabetes that you can start applying to your daily life. You will find all the information you need on moving forward with your life after you've been diagnosed, from learning what to eat and what changes to make in your diet, to finding an exercise plan you can live with, to enlisting support from your friends and family. I've included sections on working well with your doctor and information on the medical tests that you will be given. I've also included in individual chapters moments for you to reflect and look inward—a welcome opportunity, and sometimes a necessity, when one is going through life-altering times. What should a person with diabetes eat and why, what kind of exercises can I do, how can I get comfortable testing my blood glucose levels, and how can I keep healthy are all questions that will be explored in part 2. Read this and it will give you a program to work from. You'll learn how to enjoy meals outside of your home and still maintain your goals. There is a chapter on the importance of maintaining a group of caring individuals around you in all parts of your life. Alternative therapies are reviewed as an integrative approach to care. Chapter 11, "Pampering as Medicine," will inspire you to be good to yourself.

Dive in, get the information you need and use it to make your life even better than it was before you were diagnosed. The worst that can happen to you is that you will achieve some portion of the goals you have set. This book provides you with many ways of feeling like you are "winning" at diabetes. Even if it means just thinking about things you've never thought of before, or once in a while having a little bit of humor over the condition we find ourselves in, I hope that you will find this book has contributed to your living well with diabetes.

part one

Learning about Diabetes

CHAPTER 1

What Is Diabetes?

Type 2 diabetes is a chronic disorder characterized by elevated levels of glucose (sugar) in the blood. You are most likely reading this book because you have been diagnosed with type 2 diabetes, suspect you might have it, or know that a loved one has it. You are not alone. There are somewhere between 16 and 20 million people in the United States afflicted with diabetes, according to Dr. Gerald Bernstein, former president of the American Diabetes Association, although the official count has not been updated in several years. About one third of those millions are undiagnosed.

The very fact that you picked up this book and are aware of the problem of diabetes means that you are on the road to controlling it. And it can be controlled. Type 2 diabetes is so intertwined with lifestyle that it is almost impossible to discuss it without talking about the management of what you eat and the kind of exercise you get. Educate yourself and then you can use your diagnosis as an opportunity to wake up to the needs of your body, as well as your mind and spirit.

Throughout the book, you'll be given useful information to understand the physical processes that occur with diabetes.

People differ in the ways they deal with health issues—which one describes you? Some people are naturally curious about what is happening to their bodies. They visit their doctor every year and stay current with the latest medical news. And then there are people who are so busy with daily life that they don't often think about their health unless some medical problem hits them directly. These are the people who only go to the doctor if they are dragged, and rarely take a sick day even if they have the flu and a 103° temperature!

Well, to both types of people, this is your book. For the first kind, you will hopefully be interested in what is happening to your body and eagerly pursue the advice set forth within these pages. To the second set of people, this is, now more than ever before, the time when you must take notice of what is going on inside of you, so you can keep that engine running smoothly.

Your first step in dealing positively with this disease is to learn something about it. With this knowledge, diabetes is no longer a mystery that you can't explain to your loved ones. The information in this chapter will assist you in understanding the steps that you need to take to live well with this disease.

Real Lessons on Nutrients and Diabetes

Educating yourself about diabetes can require time and effort, but understanding it can provide you with the self-management to take control of blood sugars. Diabetes is a complex disease that affects your body on a variety of levels. The scientific community is always at work gathering data on causes, risk factors, and prevention. Take the time here to read about the processes that occur in your body when you are healthy and when you have diabetes. I have broken the information down into easy steps to follow so you can learn about how your body reacts to the food you consume—the type and amount of nutrients affects your everyday life by affecting your mood, your weight, your energy, and, now, your diabetes.

How Food Becomes Energy

Getting sufficient energy for the body from the food we eat is a daily pursuit—and for the senses, a pleasure. But how does the body convert food into energy? How does the cereal we eat for breakfast provide us with the power we need to function during the day, or at least until lunch?

After a meal, the body digests the food we eat. The goal of digestion is to break food down into the smallest components so that the nutrients can be released and absorbed. This is a process that begins in the mouth as we chew and ends in the small intestine with the absorption of foods' nutrients into the blood. Carbohydrates are one of the most important nutrients; they are released into the bloodstream as glucose, a simple sugar that provides for brain and nerve function and physical activity. Some glucose can be stored in the liver and muscles to be used as the body needs it. The liver, an organ in front of the stomach, is responsible for regulating storage and releasing it when needed into the bloodstream to be carried throughout our body by arteries, veins, and capillaries, and eventually to our cells. Cells, which make up our entire body, are dependent on glucose to function.

The cells throughout the body are like furnaces that need fuel every minute of every day. Imagine that the tiny molecules of glucose in the blood are the coal keeping that furnace (the cells) filled with fuel. Asleep or awake, the body is functioning constantly and it requires energy to do that: the heart beats, the brain receives and delivers messages, and muscles support the skeleton. The cells require glucose to perform, and there are several regulatory systems in our body that control how much glucose is circulated in our blood.

The Role of the Pancreas and Insulin

The pancreas is an organ behind the stomach that is the regulator of glucose in our bloodstream. Inside the pancreas there are small clusters of special cells called islets of Langerhans. That's where insulin is produced.

Insulin's job is to signal the small receptors that are present in cells to open so that they can receive glucose and thus get fueled. As the cells burn the glucose, the levels of glucose circulating in the blood, and the levels of insulin, decrease. The cycle begins again when the body detects we need more fuel and insulin levels rise to accommodate this.

When the Process Breaks Down

Sometimes the fuel that you are giving your body doesn't get absorbed. This can occur in two ways. Either the cells' receptor sites do not open when signaled by insulin or else there are too few receptors on the cells to allow the glucose to enter. As the cells fail to open to let the fuel in, glucose is built up in the blood. The pancreas knows that the cells aren't getting fed, so it keeps adding insulin into the blood. The result is that the cells experience a kind of starvation even though there is a veritable banquet on the other side of the door.

> Glucose, which is the most essential form of sugar, is also referred to as blood sugar or blood glucose. In the body, glucose = blood glucose = blood sugar, and they can all be referred to interchangeably.

When the glucose does not get absorbed, it flows into the kidneys as a waste product and gets passed out of the body in your urine. This increases urination and causes thirst. (The kidneys are a pair of organs that filter impurities from the blood and out to the bladder.) The body does not get its fuel, calls for more food, causing increased hunger, and starts to suffer from its absence, causing fatigue.

Why Does the Process Break Down?

Insulin Resistance

Many people have the genetic predisposition to develop diabetes. This may be translated into insulin resistance. This means that cells sometimes would take up the call to open from the insulin circulating in your blood and sometimes would not. As a result, your body then pumps extra insulin through your bloodstream, not knowing that there is still the initial lot of insulin that hasn't been utilized. The excess amount of insulin in your blood can be damaging to your cardiovascular system (the heart and blood vessels), causing a greater risk of heart disease.

Another damaging aspect to insulin resistance is what happens to the dietary fat you consume. Fat, found in many types of foods, needs insulin in order to shuttle it and break it down into the cells. When your cells are insulin resistant, the fat does not totally go into the cells; it continues to get pumped through the blood and eventually builds up along the walls of your veins and arteries, which can produce problems such as heart disease. Insulin resistance causes damage to the body, and should be paid attention to with the same sort of lifestyle changes recommended throughout this book.

People can move from insulin resistance to developing type 2 diabetes due to genetics and, most importantly, lifestyle practices. Different organs in the body can cause the progression from insulin resistance to type 2 diabetes. The liver may be producing too much glucose. The pancreas may be sending too little insulin into the blood. The cell receptors may not be functioning properly so that the glucose is not accepted. And of course, all this can be exacerbated by poor food choices and a lack of exercise that will lead to obesity, a risk factor for diabetes.

> You may hear the term *syndrome X* to describe the cluster of risk factors, including hypertension and elevated blood cholesterol levels, that together represent a major cause of heart disease. Insulin resistance is one of these risk factors. Often the terms *syndrome X* and *insulin resistance,* as well as *metabolic syndrome,* are used interchangeably.

The Role of Fat and Other Risk Factors in Developing Diabetes

So why does the body stop behaving itself and get diabetes? Well, one of the reasons comes from the natural aging process. This process determines that after about the age of 40 our metabolism begins to slow down, we start losing muscle mass, our hormone activity decreases, and often our physical activity levels slow down incrementally. Weight is gained more easily. For many people, weight collects around the stomach, resulting in an "apple-shaped figure." That fat, and the slow-down of physical activity, sets off a chain of reactions in the body that can increase insulin resistance. The greater the degree of obesity, the greater the degree of insulin resistance.

Fat around the middle sits right on your organs, such as the heart, lungs, stomach, kidneys, and liver, and puts pressure on them. One way to visualize this is to think of how a pregnant woman becomes increasingly uncomfortable the bigger the baby gets in her uterus—as the baby grows it pushes up the lungs and the stomach, making it harder to breathe and digest comfortably, and it constricts the intestines, and the bladder has constant pressure on it. While fat does not grow and impair the organs in such an obvious way that a baby does, it can very much hinder what's going on with organ function. Think of how difficult it is to move comfortably the bigger you are. Think of how it becomes harder to breathe. And think of all the pressure the fat is putting on your system. Your body has to work harder to function. The larger you become, the further the capillaries have to travel in order to deliver blood to your entire body.

Fat resting in your middle provides for the ready access of fat to travel to those organs, thus impeding their activity. The fat that is present in your blood requires insulin to get absorbed into your cells, and if you are insulin resistant, the fat does not settle. If your fat does not get into the cells, then it cannot be burned, and therefore it builds up in the blood. As the blood full of fatty particles circulates it can clog your arteries and lead to cardiovascular disease.

The following are some of the risk factors that can contribute to your developing diabetes. Some are in your control, like exercising regularly, and others are not, such as having a history of diabetes in your family. Because you are reading this book, you may already know that you have diabetes. But be sure to learn the risk factors for those around you, especially your close relatives who may be at risk for the disease, and friends and colleagues who may have risk factors similar to yours. Encourage them to be tested for diabetes if you think they are at risk.

In addition to being overweight or obese (see Body Mass Index chart), over 45, and not exercising enough, here are some additional risk factors for developing type 2 diabetes:

- Having a close relative with diabetes, which indicates a genetic predisposition to diabetes
- Being a woman who has given birth to a child weighing 9 pounds or more and has had complications such as frequent miscarriage, premature delivery, or toxemia
- Being a woman who has had gestational diabetes
- Having hypertension
- Triglyceride levels over 250 mg/dl
- Being of African American, Hispanic, Native American, or Asian descent

Being obese presents an individual with a five times greater risk of contracting type 2 diabetes than for someone of a healthy normal weight.

Measuring Your Body Mass Index (BMI)

Your body mass index (BMI) is a measurement used to calculate your weight as a health factor. It has been shown that as your BMI rises so does your risk for diabetes, hypertension, heart disease, and other health problems. BMI is your weight (in kilograms) divided by your height (in meters) squared.

$$BMI = \frac{weight\ (kg)}{height\ (m)2}$$

As most of us don't measure our weight in kilograms or our height in meters, multiply your weight by 703 and then divide it by your height (in inches) squared.

If you don't have a calculator, use the chart below. The left-hand side of the chart shows height. Find yours and move across to locate

WHAT'S YOUR BMI?											
Height	Body Mass Index										
	19	20	21	22	23	24	25	26	27	28	29	30
	Weight (pounds)										
4'10"	91	96	100	105	110	115	119	124	129	134	138	143
4'11"	94	99	104	109	114	119	124	128	133	138	143	148
5'0"	97	102	107	112	118	123	128	133	138	143	148	153
5'1"	100	106	111	116	122	127	132	137	143	148	153	158
5'2"	104	109	115	120	126	131	136	142	147	153	158	164
5'3"	107	113	118	124	130	135	141	146	152	158	163	169
5'4"	110	116	122	128	134	140	145	151	157	163	169	174
5'5"	114	120	126	132	138	144	150	156	162	168	174	180
5'6"	118	124	130	136	142	148	155	161	167	173	179	186
5'7"	121	127	134	140	146	153	159	166	172	178	185	191
5'8"	125	131	138	144	151	158	164	171	177	184	190	197
5'9"	128	135	142	149	155	162	169	176	182	189	196	203
5'10"	132	139	146	153	160	167	174	181	188	195	202	207
5'11"	136	143	150	157	165	172	179	186	193	200	208	215
6'0"	140	147	154	162	169	177	184	191	199	206	213	221
6'1"	144	151	159	166	174	182	189	197	204	212	219	227
6'2"	148	155	163	171	179	186	194	202	210	218	225	233
6'3"	152	160	168	176	184	192	200	208	216	224	232	240
6'4"	156	163	172	180	189	197	205	213	221	230	238	246

Source: World Health Organization

your weight. From there look up and you will find your BMI. Example: a woman who is 5 feet 5 inches tall and weighs 174 pounds has a BMI of 29 and is considered overweight.

BMI of less than 20 is considered underweight
BMI between 20 and 24 is considered desirable
BMI between 25 and 29 is considered overweight
BMI of greater than 29 is considered obese

Body mass index does not show how fit you are or where your weight is carried. Those with "apple shapes," or weight in the central part of their body, have a greater risk of heart disease, high blood pressure, and diabetes than pear-shaped people who carry their weight in the hips and thighs.

Symptoms of Type 2 Diabetes

Bonnie, fit and 54, was tired. What began as a need to rest on the weekends became a full-scale battle to get through the workweek. Her solution to this loss of energy? Lots of sugar. Milk shakes, ice cream, candy bars for a mid-morning snack. Bonnie thought that some extra-quick fuel would perk her up. The opposite occurred. She found herself becoming more and more exhausted until the day was measured by when she could get back into bed. When she began losing weight rapidly, having unquenchable thirst, and making many nighttime trips to the bathroom, she knew it was time to go to her doctor. There was no mistake about it: the symptoms equaled type 2 diabetes.

There are any number of ways that people discover they have diabetes, especially because there are so many different symptoms. Sometimes the onset is so gradual you don't even recognize that you are feeling badly. Maybe a few things have been nagging you, but nothing so severe as to send you rushing to see your doctor. So you may have only discovered it during a routine physical, like I did. Or, you may have seen your doctor because of some unusual symptoms.

Here are some of the common symptoms for type 2 diabetes that you may or may not have noticed:

- Fatigue and/or weakness
- Irritability

- Increased urination, especially causing you to awake in the middle of the night
- Increased thirst
- Increased hunger
- Weight loss or gain
- Higher occurrence than normal of colds and infections
- Longer healing time for scrapes, cuts, and bruises
- Tingling or numbness in hands and feet
- Blurry vision
- Impotence in men, lack of menstruation in women

Many people don't notice any of these symptoms, as they happen so gradually that you just get used to them. You may live with the disease from 7 to 10 years before you finally are diagnosed.

More Serious Signs of Diabetes

Hopefully, your diabetes was picked up in the early stages of its onset. If it was not, you probably were diagnosed with it because of one of the major complications that result from having diabetes, such as kidney disease, nerve disease, heart disease, or stroke. Sadly, more than half of the people with diabetes have already suffered serious damage to their systems by the time they are diagnosed. Diabetes can be a silent disease. Many people have it for years without ever recognizing it. The damage can be slow and progressive, affecting every cell in the body. It can change the very nature of the way we see, touch, move, and thus, age.

Sometimes the signs of the ravages of diabetes can be found right in front of us, but we aren't caring for ourselves in a manner that makes us mindful of some serious changes happening in our bodies. A small cut on the leg can grow into a large ulcer and remain unchecked until it becomes a major infection requiring surgery—or worse, gangrene and amputation. A slight, lingering chest pain can be a sign of angina or a heart attack. Blurred vision may be a sign that your blood sugar is out of control, or could be the first sign of retinopathy.

Chapter 2 will spell out the many complications of diabetes and how to watch for them and cope with them. Later in the book, in chapter 7, you'll get some advice on how to help make sure you stay healthy and prevent any additional complications from developing. The most important thing to remember is to be mindful of the changes that are occurring in your body. This sounds easier than it seems. For example, did you ever drive your car and not remember how you got to your destination? We can be so overworked, stressed, and bombarded with so much in life that we are listening to everything except our bodies. So be aware of any changes in your eyesight or your teeth and gums, or if you have shortness of breath, sores that don't heal, or changes in urinary habits.

Even if you have suffered from a complication of diabetes, it is not too late to start making positive changes that will help your health significantly from this moment on. It's never too late to alter your lifestyle—no matter what stage of diabetes you are in. Any modification in diet or physical activity can have an effect on the progression of diabetes. But the first step is to assess where you are now, and then create a strategy for the future.

How Type 2 Diabetes Is Diagnosed

The tests for type 2 diabetes are simple and accurate. During your yearly checkup (and I urge you and your loved ones to have one) your doctor will have a routine blood screening done. This is analyzed for a number of factors including cholesterol levels and the amount of sugar in your blood. This is called a nonfasting plasma glucose test. If you have 200 mg/dl (milligrams per deciliter) of glucose in your blood then this is a sign you may have diabetes. You may have some of the risk factors listed previously and you may have a variety of symptoms. It's also possible to be asymptomatic as many people are during the early stages of diabetes.

During my routine exam, my nonfasting plasma glucose was slightly over 200. My doctor called me to tell me the news and suggested I take four weeks to try and get my weight down and start exercising more. A month later, I had a fasting plasma glucose test. For that test, I was told to fast from after dinner until my office visit the next morning. At that time, my doctor took another blood sample and had it analyzed. When the results were returned, sure enough I had type 2 diabetes. My glucose level was 150 mg/dl.

If you take a fasting plasma glucose test and it yields a number of 126 mg/dl, it indicates diabetes. (This is a change from previous classifications, which listed the diagnosis as being at 140 mg/dl.)

You may have heard of another test called an oral glucose tolerance test, which is not often used anymore. A patient is given concentrated glucose to drink and during a three-hour period is tested to see how the blood sugar level reacts. A glucose value of 200 mg/dl or greater indicates diabetes.

After any of these tests a doctor will often urge a patient to try to lose some weight and return in a month to six weeks to be retested. If the blood sugar is still elevated, then the diagnosis is certain.

The Types of Diabetes

It's good to know about the different types of diabetes that are diagnosed, as friends, family, and colleagues will have a befuddled look on their faces when you say that you have "type 2 diabetes." What exactly does that mean, and how are the different diabetes similar and dissimilar?

Type 1

This is also called insulin-dependent diabetes and used to be called juvenile diabetes. Type 1 often occurs in people under 35, and is most commonly diagnosed in childhood or adolescence. It is an autoimmune disease, meaning that the body perceives something in the body and attacks it as an outsider or germ. In this case, pancreatic cells that produce insulin are destroyed by the body. Five to 10 percent of diabetes sufferers have this type of diabetes. In the case of type 1, insulin injections are always required to keep healthy.

Type 2

Type 2 diabetes (also known as adult onset or non–insulin dependent diabetes) is the most common type of diabetes. It makes up 90 to 95 percent of all diabetes cases. Type 2 diabetes is genetically predisposed. African Americans and Hispanics suffer almost twice as much from type 2 diabetes as Caucasians do (see chapter 3, page 46). But lifestyle plays a significant part in whether or not the disease will develop. While many need oral medications to control diabetes, changes in eating and exercise can make a significant difference in controlling this disease.

Gestational

This type of diabetes occurs solely because of pregnancy and will disappear after the pregnancy is complete. During pregnancy, the placenta produces large amounts of a variety of hormones, some of which can cause insulin resistance in the mother. Coupled with weight gain, the insulin resistance is further exacerbated. Most signs of gestational diabetes appear in the third trimester of pregnancy, although some doctors believe it is a slow, steady development throughout pregnancy that is evident by this time. If gestational diabetes is present, the pregnancy is at an increased risk for complications such as high blood pressure, preeclampsia (a severe form of edema), or fluid retention. Gestational diabetes needs to be monitored frequently and treated with diet and possibly insulin to control blood sugar levels. Gestational diabetes is a rare occurrence in pregnancy; 3 to 12 percent of women develop it, but having it once will increase your risk for it recurring in later pregnancies and puts you at increased risk (nearly 40 percent) for developing type 2 diabetes later on. There is some evidence that shows the same genes that contribute to type 2 diabetes are in evidence in gestational diabetes. It occurs more frequently in older women and in the high-risk groups of African Americans, Hispanic Americans, Native Americans, and some Asian Americans and Pacific Islanders. Obesity is also associated with high risk for having gestational diabetes.

Others
Instances of diabetes may occur from genetic defects, surgery, drugs, malnutrition, infections, and other illnesses, and account for 1 to 2 percent of all diagnosed cases of diabetes. The use of protease inhibitors for patients with AIDS has been known to cause diabetes. Some think it has to do with the medications, which can tax the liver and kidneys.

What Can You Do about This Disease?

Diabetes is a chronic disease, meaning that, unless they find a cure, you will live with it for the rest of your life. But there is much that can be done to help you live well with this disease. For instance, you should eat a healthy diet, try to lose weight if you are overweight, exercise, monitor your blood sugar frequently to stay at a controlled level, and get the support you need with these efforts from your friends, family, and colleagues.

These changes to your life require a lot of work, vigilance, and ongoing education. In fact, with diabetes, you may feel like you are back in school or in a foreign country with a new language and customs. It can be disorienting. Words and concepts will be new to you, and you will begin to redefine priorities in your life. It's the goal of this book to give you useful information that will assist you in managing your diabetes. Get the facts. Continue to read this book and understand the ramifications of your diagnosis—and the lifestyle decisions available to you. The next chapter is on all of the complications that can happen to you with diabetes. You can help to avoid them if you make real changes to your life today.

CHAPTER 2

Diabetes: The Toll It Takes

U ncle Shaya was an amputee. He had one leg and used a crutch to get around. Shaya was my Grandma Beckie's brother. They both had diabetes, but I didn't know that growing up. I thought Uncle Shaya must have lost his leg in "The War." In the '50s, it seemed that most hardships had something to do with World War II, so I couldn't imagine that a family gene or lifestyle would cause Shaya to lose a leg. It seemed so much more imaginable to me that an enemy out there somewhere caused all this hardship, and not something from within.

It's often difficult to imagine what all the implications are to your life when you are first diagnosed with diabetes. You think: Can this be happening to me? And then you start to think about the complications associated with diabetes. You may have thoughts about family members with diabetes who have had amputations, lost their sight, or had a heart attack. So consciously or unconsciously, that may be in the back of your mind as you confront your own diagnosis. You may refuse to think about complications. Unfortunately, this denial can have huge consequences. Every year, over 190,000 Americans die of diabetes and its complications.

My mother, who was diagnosed about 20 years ago, has retinopathy. Her vision has gotten progressively worse and one of her simple joys, reading, has become a challenge. When I asked her how she felt about it she said, "I never took diabetes seriously until it hurt my vision." How many of us are in that place?

It's difficult to come to grips with a disease that can be "silent" for years. Yet by the time it progresses, there's no denying its effects. Heart disease, kidney failure, or even amputation can result from ignoring the disease. My mother says she is in such denial she wishes she had a bucket of sand to put her head in. When I tell her about my own fears, she says, "Wait, I'll lend you my bucket of sand!" That's not going to work for me.

It's important to take a deep breath and understand what the complications of diabetes are and how they need to be treated. To be an informed diabetes patient, you should understand what is happening in your body. Educate yourself with this chapter about what diabetes can do—the effects, over time, can be very far-reaching and debilitating. I urge you to take the steps necessary to take care of yourself. Think about all the things you want to do with the rest of your life—time spent with loved ones, grandchildren, travel, learning, and just plain old relaxing. If you start making changes in your life today with the advice that follows in part 2, it will affect your health for the better now and in the future.

The Importance of Tight Control

You may hear from your doctors, in the news, and throughout this book the importance of controlling your blood sugar. Sometimes you may question why this is so important, especially when you may not be experiencing many symptoms of your diabetes, and complications seem like a distant issue. Well, in 1993, research was released from a pivotal 10-year study called DCCT (Diabetes Control and Complications). Although the study focused on type 1, doctors have seen the significance for type 2: by maintaining tight control of blood glucose levels a marked decrease in micro (neuropathies) and macro (heart disease) complications can occur.

More recently the United Kingdom Prospective Diabetes Study (UKPDS) of 5,000 subjects further emphasized these findings for type 2. *The key message was that to reduce complications it is essential to control blood glucose levels, HbA1c levels, and blood pressure.* This was emphasized to me when I interviewed Dr. Robin Goland, the director of the Naomi Berrie Diabetes Center at Columbia-Presbyterian Hospital. Dr. Goland stressed the importance of keeping control of blood glucose levels because it can make a difference in keeping at bay micro vascular complications.

What Diabetes Can Do to Your Body

Having the high blood sugar levels that are associated with unchecked diabetes damages your blood vessels. That concentrated amount of glucose running through your veins causes the small blood vessels to become brittle. Blood then has a harder time getting through the thickened vessel walls. This in turn causes a lack of feeling in different parts of your body. Usually limbs are the first to experience this because they are the farthest from the heart and have some very tiny vessels. That's why we often experience numbness in our feet and fingers. In addition, the blood vessels in your heart, kidneys, and eyes can become damaged.

Diabetes is often called an aging disease because of the strain it puts on so many organs and systems. This premature aging can occur as your small blood vessels and many of your organs, including your heart and kidneys, are taxed by the struggle of operating with an impaired system. The effects of this struggle can be as minor as the feeling of pins and needles in your extremities or as dramatic as kidney failure. Many of the major complications can be prevented, or their progression can be stopped, by paying attention to them at their earliest stages.

Different Types of Diabetes-Related Complications

In this section, we will explore many of the complications that can result from diabetes. Each complication has a brief description of what can happen to the body from diabetes, what the symptoms are, and how the disease can be treated. Think of it as an overview of what can happen, what to look out for, when to call your doctor, and what kind of treatment can be expected. Consult your health professionals today if you suspect you are suffering from one of these complications.

Cardiovascular Disease

Research has shown that people with diabetes have a far greater number of cardiovascular complications than those without, and the chance of death from cardiovascular disease is two to four times as likely. Women with type 2 are at particular risk. They are three to four times more likely to have cardiovascular disease than women without diabetes.

Heart disease accounts for 40 percent of all deaths of people with diabetes. Hypertension is the single most important factor leading to a stroke.

What happens to your heart? Your heart is a muscle pumping blood throughout your body. The arteries and capillaries carry blood away from your heart and to your body, and veins carry the blood back to your heart. Diabetes can affect your heart by increasing your triglyceride levels, and by disrupting the activities of and sometimes the ratios between "good" and "bad" cholesterol. These effects can cause a hardening of the arteries known as atherosclerosis. This is a type of very hard plaque that is built up in your blood vessels, clogging and narrowing the space in which your blood can be moved through to the rest of your body and back to your heart. Diabetes patients also tend to get heart disease because many times they have the additional risk factors of eating high-fat foods and leading a sedentary lifestyle. The life plan in this book will help you turn around those factors, and help you lower your cholesterol, so your risk of developing cardiovascular disease is lowered.

Cardiovascular disease may manifest itself in the following ways:

Hypertension (High Blood Pressure)

Hypertension refers to the high pressure at which your blood is flowing through your veins and arteries. Narrowed blood vessels can cause high blood pressure, as the force is greater when the blood has to travel through a smaller space. Obesity and kidney problems can also contribute to high blood pressure.

High blood pressure can be measured very easily and quickly in the doctor's office or even at home with a home blood pressure monitor. You will see or be given two numbers that tell you your blood pressure. The first number, the top number, is the systolic pressure. This should be under 130 for normal readings. The second (bottom) number is the diastolic pressure, which should read about 80. Talk to your physician about what a goal blood pressure is for you.

 Warning Signs of Severe High Blood Pressure

Most people don't know they have high blood pressure until they have theirs read at the doctor's office. But there are emergency symptoms that you should know about:

- Bad headache
- Irritability
- Confusion
- Episode of fainting
- Loss of vision
- Chest pain
- Shortness of breath
- Numbness or weakness in a limb

Seek emergency medical attention if you experience these symptoms.

Treatment

Reducing your blood pressure involves many of the elements suggested in this book, such as improving your diet, losing weight, and exercising more. If you do have high blood pressure, it is important to reduce your sodium/salt intake to 2,000 mg a day. In addition, increasing your potassium, calcium, and magnesium may help to reduce blood pressure. You can do this by increasing your intake of fruits, vegetables, and low-fat dairy products like milk and yogurt. However, take note of the carbohydrate content in fruit and milk products to keep your blood sugar under control.

There are many medications used to treat high blood pressure that you will likely get prescribed, including: diuretics, beta-blockers, alpha receptor agonists, alpha-blockers, direct blood vessel dilators, ACE inhibitors, and calcium channel blockers.

Angina (Chest Pain)

Angina is chest pain, but it can also be felt in the arms, shoulders, neck, jaw, and back. As the blood vessels narrow due to plaque formation, the heart does not receive enough oxygen carried by the blood and angina occurs. The pain results from a lack of oxygen to the heart. When your energy requirements go up, for example during stressful occasions or during exercise, the heart works so hard that it needs more and more oxygen to keep working. However, sufficient oxygen cannot get to the heart because of narrowed blood vessels and lactic acid builds up causing angina. But when you calm down, or stop exercising, the heart can get enough oxygen and the pain goes away.

Angina, therefore, is a warning sign that your heart is having trouble doing its job, and you need to stop immediately whatever is working your heart up—whether it be having an argument with a mate, some sort of exercise, or a generally stressful situation. Seek help for your angina, as without treatment for your heart, you may have a heart attack. Angina is often a signal that a person may be having a heart attack or may have a heart attack within weeks, months, or years.

Treatment

Angina is often treated with nitroglycerin to relieve the pain. A person with angina will be taught what to do and how to use the medication in case of an attack.

Heart Attack

A heart attack, known medically as a myocardial infarction (MI), is the loss of part of the heart muscle due to lack of blood flow. This can occur either through the narrowing of an artery to the extent that it becomes blocked or when a piece of plaque that has been building up on your veins or arteries becomes dislodged from the wall and gets lodged somewhere narrow, stopping or reducing blood flow.

Warning Signs of a Heart Attack

- Pain: a squeezing or crushing pain beneath your breast bone, in the left side of the chest, and going to the arm, neck, jaw, or throat.
- Indigestion pain
- Clamminess, sweating
- Nausea and/or vomiting
- Shortness of breath
- Weakness
- Near-fainting or fainting

Note: 25 percent of people who have had a heart attack do not experience these symptoms, and women may experience different symptoms, such as pain that is not centered in the chest, nausea or dizziness without pain, and more. Especially with diabetes and the damage that may have been done to your nerves, you may not feel that you are having a heart attack, but if you notice any ill feelings, report it to your doctor.

If you think you are experiencing a heart attack, call 911 or have someone do it for you. Do not think that you are acting brave if you ignore it, even if you only have some of the symptoms. The faster you can get help, the faster your heart muscle will be saved, increasing your odds of survival and having a longer and more comfortable life span. If you live in a rural area and it would take time for an ambulance to arrive, see if you can get driven to the hospital quickly. Lie down, try to stay calm, and take long, deep breaths. Talk to your physician about what to do if any of these symptoms occur. At such times people are often told to take a regular aspirin, which will help the blood not to clot. Make sure to keep aspirin in the house in case of such an emergency. More than 20 percent of people suffering a heart attack die before reaching the hospital (usually in the first hour). Rapid treatment can cut this number in half.

> Every day approximately 350 people with diabetes die of a heart attack. Seventy-five percent of people with diabetes will die from heart attacks or strokes in the U.S. —*Centers for Disease Control (CDC)*

Treatment

In the emergency room, the doctors will try to ease your pain and anxiety with drugs and oxygen, while determining if you have had a heart attack. If they do make that determination, they will likely give you "clot-busting" drugs to dissolve the blood clot.

Later, you may be given a balloon angioplasty to open your clogged artery or have bypass surgery. An angioplasty also is done when lifestyle changes, such as diet and exercise, and medication fail to help angina pain. It is performed usually under local anesthetic, and can be done in as little as an hour. This is usually the preferred method of treatment, if your cardiologist thinks you are a candidate for the surgery, as it is less invasive and requires much less recovery time and expense than bypass surgery.

Bypass Surgery

Bypass surgery "bypasses" blocked or narrowed arteries by using healthy veins or arteries, taken from your own body, and inserting them into the coronary artery or arteries. This ensures good blood flow to the heart. As many as five "detours" may be done in your heart. This is a major surgical procedure, and the risk of the surgery climbs with diabetes, kidney disease, and age. If a damaging lifestyle is continued with high-fat food, smoking, and little exercise, it's likely that those new arteries will become clogged too.

After a Heart Attack

When you are discharged from the hospital, you will probably need to take medications to prevent more clots from forming, which can include such drugs as aspirin, beta-blockers, or digitalis. You may eventually require surgery to help fix or bypass blocked arteries. Recovery will take about six weeks, depending on your degree of heart attack and type of treatment. Follow the advice in chapter 7, Taking Care of Yourself, to help prevent future heart attacks.

Stroke

Stroke has often been referred to as a "brain attack," because, like a heart attack, the oxygen is not flowing to the brain because of a clogged vein or artery and the brain starts to die. The same plaque that can cause a heart attack can also clog the arteries that go to the brain. Another cause of a stroke can be when a piece of plaque breaks off of a vein or artery and ends up lodged and stuck in one of the brain's blood vessels. Yet another cause can be when an artery to the brain bursts, from either high blood pressure or weakened walls.

Cells deprived of oxygen start dying rapidly. The longer the brain is deprived of oxygen, the more damage is done, and a lot of it is permanent. Just as angina is a sign of coronary artery disease and may precede a heart attack, sometimes (10 percent of the time) people have temporary but transient symptoms of impending strokes. Known as transient ischemic attacks—TIAs—these symptoms need your doctor's immediate attention so that he or she may prevent you from having a stroke.

Warning Signs of a Stroke

- Numbness or weakness in one side of the body
- Loss or partial loss of vision in one eye
- Trouble talking or comprehending speech
- Severe headache
- Dizziness or falls

Call 911 or have yourself driven to a hospital immediately if you experience signs of a stroke. As with a heart attack, the faster you receive treatment, the more the risk of devastating damage and death declines.

Treatment

Doctors need to determine the cause of stroke in order to start treatment. This is usually done by viewing a CT scan of the brain. One of the big concerns with treating a stroke is not only to stop it from further damaging your brain, but also to make sure the treatment itself doesn't cause further damage. Eighty percent of all strokes are ischemic, which means they result from clogged arteries or a blood clot. The administration of a drug called tissue plasminogen activator (tPA), which is also used to dissolve clots in heart attacks, can be given within three hours of the first signs of stroke if an ischemic stroke is determined to have taken place. It cannot be given in all cases, but it is good to know about. Your doctors must first determine that you are having an ischemic attack, because if you are experiencing bleeding in your brain because of an embolism and a clot-busting drug is given, your brain could bleed further and cause massive problems.

If your carotid artery is partially blocked, you may be a candidate for carotid endarterectomy. The carotid arteries are the arteries that flow through the sides of your neck, supplying blood to your brain. If one is blocked, there is an operation that can be done that removes the plaque from that artery to give a clear path for the blood to flow. Tens of thousands of these operations are performed every year.

In the case of a brain hemorrhage, where a vessel bursts in your brain, the bleeding must be controlled. Half of all people die because of the pressure on the brain.

The results of a stroke can be anywhere from minor to major. Physical skills can be lost, parts of the body can be paralyzed, and speech may be affected. Rehabilitation may be necessary to relearn lost skills.

 The chances of a stroke are the same for men and women. All people with diabetes are two to four times more likely to have a stroke as those without.

A Note about Smoking

Cigarette smoking produces additional risks for heart disease in everyone, and it is particularly dangerous for people with diabetes. If you smoke, make every effort to stop now. Speak with your doctor about smoking cessation programs, nicotine patches, and behavior modification.

Retinopathy and Other Eye Damage

Causes

Diabetes is the leading cause of blindness. Each year as many as 24,000 Americans lose their sight because of diabetes. Nearly half of all people who have diabetes will eventually have some form of eye disease, usually diabetic retinopathy. Hypertension adds an additional risk factor for retinopathy. But many problems can be averted if dealt with quickly, and damage can be kept to a minimum. It's often dependent on the control of blood sugar. However, more than 60 percent of people with type 2 will have some retinopathy after 20 years.

Because retinopathy can progress for many years without symptoms, yearly dilated eye exams with an ophthalmologist or optometrist experienced in diabetes care is essential.

As with other complications listed here, retinopathy begins with damage to the blood vessels, in this case, in your eyes. The back of the eye, where light is reflected and images are processed, is called the retina. Tiny blood vessels in the retina can weaken and leak. As the disease progresses, new blood vessels can form on the retina, and these can bleed, cloud vision, and, eventually, destroy it.

Nonproliferative retinopathy is the most common form of retinopathy, and in many cases it does not impact vision. The capillaries that provide blood to the retina form pouches but do not leak. It has little to no effect on vision and usually needs no treatment. However, if leakage or fluid in the central area of the eye (the macula) does occur it may diminish light in the eye and affect vision. This is called macular edema. It may be mild and require little attention. But this disease can progress and cause lesions in the eye, developing into proliferative retinopathy. As the eye compensates for weakened or destroyed blood vessels, new blood vessels are formed. Unfortunately this compensation that occurs creates additional problems since the new blood vessels that grow to replace the old are too weak for their job and leak. This blocks vision, and scar tissue will form at the site of the hemorrhage. The scar tissue then may shrink as it heals, and hurt the retina even further. You may experience a floating line or web in your vision or "floaters," dark spots that appear to be swimming in front of your eyes.

Because major damage can occur before you notice any symptoms, it is imperative that you see your eye doctor for an exam at least once a year.

Warning Signs of Eye Problems
- Blurry vision
- Double vision
- Reduced eyesight or reduced peripheral vision
- Pain or pressure in the eye
- Floaters or spots in your vision

If you have blurred vision on a particular day, you can use this as a sign that you may be experiencing high glucose levels. Bring your level down and the blurred vision will go away. However, if you do not tightly control your diabetes over time, you may develop retinopathy.

Treatment

Eyes can be saved with laser treatment if the disease is caught early, before any major damage is done. The laser treatments are called photocoagulation, which seals the blood vessels to prevent them from leaking, and scatter photocoagulation, which is also used sometimes for glaucoma. Surgery is also a treatment that may be considered if the retina is detached and there is a lot of blood in the eye.

 A Note about Glaucoma
Glaucoma is caused by too much pressure building up in the eye, eventually pinching the nerves that serve the retina. Those with diabetes are nearly twice as likely to get glaucoma than those who do not have the disease. The longer you have had the disease, and the older you are, the more likely you are to be at risk.

Kidney Disease

Causes

Diabetes can cause a narrowing and weakening of small blood vessels in the kidneys, and is responsible for 40 percent of the new cases of end-stage renal disease diagnosed every year. There is no cure for diabetes-related kidney disease, which is called nephropathy. Treatment involves only trying to control and slow its progression to kidney failure. Most people do not develop a nephropathy that is severe enough to result in end-stage renal disease, which is when your kidneys can no longer do their job and must be aided by dialysis or be replaced with a healthy kidney.

The kidneys, which filter your blood, lose their efficiency with nephropathy. As such damage occurs, blood flow is increased to the kidneys and the filtration units, called glomeruli, resulting in an increase in size of both. With disease progression, the glomeruli begin to show damage, as the protein albumin leaks into the urine. Even tiny amounts can be identified by a urine test for microalbumin. This is important because albumin naturally flows throughout our bloodstream and should not be excreted in the urine. Protein in the urine can be a sign of kidney damage. In addition, as the disease progresses, the kidneys lose their ability to filter out waste products, and levels of creatinine and urea nitrogen build up in the blood. With a blood sample, your physician can monitor your kidney function. Although many people who have nephropathy never have the disease progress to end-stage, with the average time of onset being 23 years from onset of diabetes, it is critical that you take such a complication seriously and work at preventing it.

It is thought that high blood pressure may contribute to the development of kidney disease in diabetes patients and may speed up the progression of the disease. And, ironically, kidney disease can raise blood pressure, since one of the functions of the kidney is to regulate blood pressure. It is important to keep your blood pressure in check, as well as control blood sugar levels.

Warning Signs of Kidney Disease
- Leg swelling, leg cramps
- Increased need to urinate, especially at night
- Protein in the urine, occasionally detected by foamy urine
- High blood pressure
- Abnormal blood tests, such as a rise in blood urea nitrogen (BUN), and creatinine tests
- Less need for insulin or antidiabetic pills
- Morning sickness, nausea, and vomiting
- Itching

Treatment

Treatment involves controlling high blood pressure, reducing protein intake in the diet, controlling blood sugar levels, adequate fluid intake (six to eight glasses of water per day), avoiding kidney-damaging medications, and quick treatment and avoidance of urinary tract infections.

For those with kidney failure, there is the possibility of kidney transplant or dialysis, either peritoneal dialysis or hemodialysis. Dialysis is a blood-filtering process. Peritoneal dialysis can be done at home several times a day, whereas hemodialysis is usually done at a medical facility three times a week. Lastly, while kidney transplants can be performed, they are mostly recommended for diabetics under the age of 50 without any other medical complications.

Nerve Disease (Neuropathy)

Causes

Diabetic neuropathy, or nerve disease, is a complication that the majority of us may have (60 to 70 percent), but luckily only half of those who have it experience any symptoms. The longer you have had diabetes, the more likely you are to develop nerve damage.

High blood sugar is thought to be the reason for nerve damage in diabetics. The nervous system is a network that carries messages between your brain and spinal cord, on the one hand, and your muscles, skin, organs, and vessels on the other. Your nervous system helps control just about everything that your body does.

Neuropathy can manifest itself all over your body with tingling, burning, and numbness (peripheral diffuse neuropathy), or can target a specific place in your body (autonomic diffuse neuropathy).

Peripheral is the easier one to recognize. The term describes damage between nerves that convey sensations from your limbs to your brain.

 Signs of Peripheral Neuropathy

- Tingling
- Burning
- Pins and needles
- Cramping
- Numbness
- Loss of sensation
- Glove-and-stocking sensation (it feels as though you are wearing gloves and/or stockings all the time)

For many people, the disease is mild. But it must be looked after if you have a loss of sensation, because you may not feel any problems with your feet that can come from infection, or if you adopt a different type of gait that may signal muscle weakness.

Autonomic Diffuse Neuropathy

Autonomic nerves control the systems in your body that are unconsciously working, such as digestive systems, cardiovascular systems, the sex organs, the urinary tract, and how you respond to low blood sugar.

Digestive system damage could result in nausea, vomiting, diarrhea, constipation, fecal incontinence, and heartburn. If you do not digest normally, you might experience problems with hypoglycemia.

Cardiovascular damage can affect the signals that are sent regarding how much blood we need and when and blood pressure. Signs of such damage may be light-headedness because of low blood pressure, or you might have a heart attack and not know it because of the lack of nerve endings there.

Sexual organs can be affected by nerve damage and circulatory problems. This may cause impotence in men and lack of a sexual response in women.

Urinary problems can occur if the nerves around the bladder are damaged. Your bladder might not know if it's completely emptied, and frequent infections may result. Another problem might be incontinence because the bladder lacks the nerve endings to tell you that it is full.

Your sweat glands can be affected by nerve damage, and you could wake up at night drenched in sweat or not be able to cool off during a hot summer's day because of the lack of the ability of your body to recognize the need to cool itself down.

Treatment

Blood sugar control is paramount in keeping this disease from progressing, and may even relieve some symptoms. Treatment may include medications for pain relief. Apply topical cream that has capsaicin in it; this is the same ingredient that gives peppers their hotness. When applied to specific areas of neuropathy these creams can give some relief. It's important not to apply this cream to open sores.

Prevention

Damage to the nervous system cannot be reversed. The only way to prevent damage to the nervous system is to keep your blood glucose levels under as tight control as you can.

Infections

In diabetes, infections are common and varied. The abundant amount of glucose in the blood renders the white blood cells, which fight infection, less able to battle the many pathogens we are all exposed to. No matter where the site of infection, having too much glucose in your blood can affect the ability of the body to fight off bacteria, viruses, or fungi. In addition, the glucose itself becomes food for many of these pathogens to feed on. So not only can they attack more easily, they also can multiply faster. Common sites of infection are on the skin, mouth and gums, feet, and genitals. This is why it is so important to clean all sores and infections, maintain good sanitary habits, and of course, keep tight control on blood sugar.

Gum Disease

Causes

Gum disease is caused by the damage of having high blood sugar, as well as from blood vessel damage. High sugar levels in the mouth can cause bacteria to grow, and vessel damage can prevent waste products in the mouth from being taken away and nutrients from being brought to the site of the infection. Although it is quite a common problem among all adults, your chances increase of getting gum infections if you have diabetes, and especially if you have poor control over your blood glucose.

 Warning Signs of Gum Disease
- Bleeding gums when you brush or floss
- Red, swollen, or tender gums
- Gums that have pulled away from teeth
- Pus between the gums
- Bad breath
- Loose teeth

Gingivitis is an inflammation of the gums because of a buildup of plaque. It can progress to periodontitis, which is a condition characterized by a pulling away of your gums from your teeth. In that space, infected pockets form. If nothing is done, this infection will destroy your teeth. Also beware of oral infections or thrush, which is a fungal infection, resulting in white patches in your mouth, which may turn sore and make it difficult to swallow.

Diabetes patients sometimes complain about dry mouth, which may be due to certain medications. Dry mouth can increase your risk of getting gingivitis since saliva, which naturally contains antibacterial components that protect your mouth from bacterial overgrowth and infections, is lessened.

Treatment

Treatment for periodontitis depends on the severity of the infection. The infection needs to be cleaned out under the gum, and this can sometimes be accomplished by a deep cleaning. Prescribed antibiotics or mouthwashes may be needed to halt the infection. Gum surgery may be necessary, if the disease is advanced, to save teeth.

Prevention

Because it's difficult to detect the early warning signs of periodontitis, visit the dentist or periodontist at least twice a year. For a dry mouth, try chewing sugar-free gum or candy to keep the saliva flowing. Always remember to brush and floss regularly in order to control plaque, but this alone cannot prevent the spread of periodontitis once it has begun.

Skin Sores

People with diabetes are more likely to have skin infections than those who don't have diabetes. In addition to the risks from higher sugar levels and possible lower white blood cell count, poor circulation also contributes to infections. They can be either fungal, yeast, or bacterial.

Yeast infections (candida) develop in moist areas of the skin or mucous membranes. The most vulnerable are areas around the genitals, the skin inside the mouth, and around skin folds. There are topical creams often used to heal yeast infections. It's important to keep the area dry in order to avoid splitting and cracking of the skin.

Other forms of infections include open wounds, which can cause scar tissue, boils, or yellow bumps.

Foot Complications

Causes

There can be a variety of causes that lead to problems with your feet. Nerve damage, or neuropathy, can cause a loss of feeling in your feet, as well as cause burning or pain sensations. This can also cause muscle weakness in the legs and feet, foot deformities (such as hammertoes and bunions), and conditions such as blisters, corns, and calluses.

Poor circulation, from the narrowing of blood vessels, can cause cramping and pain in the legs or calves, make the feet feel constantly cold or turn them bright red, and make the skin more easily damaged as it becomes thinner. There is a loss of restorative oxygen and nutrients to flow to the feet. This loss of feeling can cause something that might once have been a minor inconvenience, such as a blister, into a serious complication. A tiny blister can get infected, end up as a wound, and, because your body no longer has the healing powers it once did (due to malfunctions in your white blood cells), might end up causing your foot to require surgery. And this horrible turn of events can come about because you couldn't feel that your shoe was rubbing up and pinching, or didn't tend to it quickly enough.

It is estimated that 15 percent of people suffering from diabetes will be hospitalized from a serious foot condition at some point during their lives. But most of the complications of diabetes-related foot problems can be prevented. A more extensive discussion of how to take care of your feet can be found in chapter 7.

Treatment

It is so important to recognize the need for early treatment of foot problems. If a wound on your foot does not start healing by your own measures in 24 hours, you must call your podiatrist immediately and start treatment. Avoid pressure on that foot until you can see the doctor.

The doctor will try to treat the wound with antibiotics and bandages, and may also try to relieve pressure on the area by making you take weight off of your foot by using a crutch, a wheelchair, or giving you special shoe inserts or casts. If your circulation is so bad that it cannot repair the wound with treatment, it may be necessary to see a vascular surgeon to try to reconstruct some of the blood vessels in your feet.

Amputation

According to the American Diabetes Association up to 85 percent of lower-extremity amputations could be avoided by improved prevention and treatment of foot ulcers and proper education about foot care.

As stated, circulation and nerve damage are complications that befall many people with diabetes. Unfortunately when these complications are unattended on legs or feet, they can lead to lower-extremity amputations. Even a simple blister or a cut on the foot that becomes infected can begin the process, especially when it was not felt due to neuropathy. As much as 50 percent of all nontraumatic lower-extremity amputations in the U.S. are from people with diabetes.

Read the information in chapter 7 for proper foot care that will assist in the prevention of amputation.

Now that we have learned about many of the complications that can afflict a person with diabetes, let's take a look at how different populations are affected by diabetes.

CHAPTER 3

How Different People Are Affected by Diabetes

D iabetes is a rising problem across all populations in the United States. Type 2 diabetes is close to being officially recognized by the government as an "epidemic" given the increasing numbers of people developing it every year. About 650,000 people are diagnosed annually. That's almost 1,800 new cases per day.

> **Get involved!** It's important, as you fight diabetes in your own body, to convey to those around you the risks of diabetes. They can take preventive steps today to avoid the disease in the future. Help stop the spread of this disease. Join the American Diabetes Association to become more involved in the battle against diabetes.

I ran a diabetes support group for New York University. There, young and old, African American and Caucasian shared the common experiences of being afflicted with diabetes. Together, we must face complications, monitor our blood sugar, eat a healthy diet, and exercise in order to keep healthy.

But there are certain differences in the way the disease affects us as groups. Certain ethnicities have a higher predisposition to type 2. For example, the African American community has nearly twice the rate of diabetes, and experiences many more serious complications, than non-Hispanic whites.

Gender also presents particular issues. For men, impotency can result from having type 2 diabetes. Pregnant women can experience gestational diabetes, which furthers the risk of type 2 in the future.

This chapter explores some of these differences and the risk factors associated with ethnicity and gender.

Women and Diabetes

Women have some particular risks and complications associated with diabetes. For example African American women, Hispanic women, and Native American women all have an increased chance of contracting the disease. If a woman has gestational diabetes during her pregnancy (see chapter 1), she has a much increased risk of getting type 2 diabetes after her pregnancy ends. Menopause can signal the onset of diabetes. For those women who already have diabetes, menopause can have a strong effect on the existing condition.

Complications for Women with Diabetes

Vaginal and Urinary Tract Infections

Women with diabetes are more prone to getting vaginal infections. High blood sugar creates an environment that fosters this and causes it to be a chronic condition. The best precaution to take is to exercise good blood glucose control. A urinary tract infection should be treated by a doctor immediately, as it could move to your kidneys, which might be weakened from diabetes already. A yeast infection can be treated with one of several effective over-the-counter medications. Of course, if this is the first time you have had a yeast infection, or if it persists, contact your doctor. Those of us with diabetes should be highly vigilant when dealing with any infection.

Sex

For the most part, women with type 2 diabetes confront the same sexual issues common to all women. However, there are certain conditions that can be exacerbated by the disease. Physical symptoms such as vaginal dryness, yeast infections, and nerve damage can decrease pleasure. These complications may not happen to every woman, but it's important to be aware of the effect they do have when they occur. When these conditions are present even the fear of the discomfort can diminish sexual desire. We also have to look at our self-image and sense of self. Do we feel less desirable or potent because of this disease? If you are experiencing any diminished desire, it's useful to take a look at these issues.

 Diabetes and Menstruation

Menstruation can affect the level of blood glucose in your body, which may rise a few days before your period begins. You may need to increase insulin to counteract this effect.

It's difficult to say whether type 2 diabetes has a direct effect on women and sex (see also under "Men"). Some of the symptoms associated with menopause and hormonal fluctuations can also account for a change in sexual desire. Talk to your gynecologist about any problems you may be having. She will be familiar with the many factors that can bring about sexual problems, and can help you with hormone replacement therapies and other remedies. The first step is to have a complete examination to make sure there aren't additional physical problems affecting your sexuality.

A Note about Birth Control

Birth control can affect diabetes control: the pill may raise your blood glucose levels and also may increase your blood pressure. Talk to your doctor about whether this form of birth control is best for you.

An IUD (intrauterine device) used for birth control can cause infections and should not be used by diabetic women.

Menopause

The onset of menopause brings its own set of issues associated with diabetes. Were you diagnosed with diabetes around the time of menopause? Many women are. This is the time when production of several of our hormones and our metabolism slow down and it becomes harder to maintain a steady weight. In fact, it's a time when many of us begin to gain weight. If we have a predisposition to diabetes it often kicks in at menopause.

It seems like so much can happen to women at about the same time in life. Some studies have indicated that menopause can occur earlier in women with type 2 diabetes (although this has been disputed). Other studies indicate that menopausal women with diabetes tend to have more emotional swings than those without diabetes and many other menopausal symptoms are worse. It's a common scenario for women to visit their doctor because of these symptoms and then be diagnosed with diabetes.

Now that I have lived through menopause and the diagnosis of diabetes, I'm not sure whether the symptoms I was suffering from were blood sugar lows or a bout of menopausal emotions.

If you were diagnosed with diabetes before menopause, you may notice that you need less insulin to keep your blood glucose levels at a normal range. That is because estrogen and progesterone actually combat insulin, and so more is usually necessary when the female hormones are actively being made. When menopause occurs and those hormones are stopped on the production line, you will notice the change in your glucose levels. That is a good enough reason to keep track of your levels at all times. However, weight gain and lack of exercise may counteract your decreasing needs for insulin by raising glucose levels again.

Often the symptoms of menopause can be confused with hypoglycemia. Symptoms of menopause can make women who have diabetes worry that they are having episodes of hypoglycemia, as they are the same symptoms (sweating, hot flashes). Women with type 2 diabetes can take hormone replacement therapy (HRT), but may have a higher incidence of endometrial cancer. Does the risk of that cancer outweigh increased risk of getting a heart attack, stroke, and all the rest of the problems associated with loss of female hormones because of diabetes? Many doctors fully believe in hormone replacement therapy. Discuss your particular pros and cons and the risks involved with your gynecologist.

Men

Men have their own problems with diabetes too. The one of biggest concern is that of erectile dysfunction. It may be erectile dysfunction that first leads a man to visit his doctor, not knowing it is an underlying condition, such as diabetes, that may be causing the problem.

Erectile dysfunction (ED), more commonly known as impotence (the inability to achieve or maintain an erection for intercourse), in men with diabetes may be over 50 percent in men over 60. ED does not mean that a man cannot attain an erection, but that the erection either cannot be sustained or is not strong enough for intercourse. This is a problem that many men face as they get older, and can occur because of a combination of events, but the incidence of this disorder can occur earlier in men with diabetes.

According to the American Diabetes Association, 8 percent of all men with type 2 diabetes have impotence.

ED in men with diabetes may be due to nerve damage or blood vessel damage, usually caused by poor blood glucose control. As an erection depends on a combination of events occurring successfully, with muscles, nerves, and blood vessels all working together, it is easy to see how one thing wrong in that combination can interfere with the process. Blood flow must be good to the penis, and a sphincter response is regulated by the nervous system. Both of these can be damaged by diabetes. The longer a man has had diabetes, the more likely it is that he may have impairment. Other complications from diabetes, such as cardiovascular problems and neuropathy, may also be contributing to ED.

Other factors, such as some medications (high blood pressure medications, beta-blockers, antidepressants), too much alcohol and cigarette consumption, stress, depression, illness, and boredom, also may be causing ED.

The many recommendations made throughout this book should help you with ED. But more specifically, the herb ginkgo is recommended as it may improve blood flow to the penis. The prescription medication Viagra may help. Couples can seek counseling to improve lovemaking and to learn new ways of making love that will relax you instead of making you feel anxious.

Children

When we think of diabetes afflicting children, most people assume that what they are suffering from is juvenile, or type 1 diabetes, a condition that plagues children and adolescents that causes the pancreas to stop producing insulin. But recently, there has been a rise in type 2 diabetes among this young population. Of the children diagnosed with diabetes, indications are that anywhere between 8 percent and 45 percent of them have type 2 diabetes, dependent upon race and ethnicity. Researchers have not been able to clarify the exact percentage since more studies need to be done in examining this new phenomenon. The main cause of the rise in type 2 diabetes in children is the rise in childhood obesity, which has become an epidemic in the United States. Puberty and racial/ethnic heritage (Hispanic, American Indian, and African American) also contribute to this growing phenomenon.

Why is this terrible disease staking a claim on the young? You can blame it on computers, remote control TV, and a lack of mandatory physical education programs in schools. Today's kids seem not to be allowed to play outside on their own for hours at a time the way we might have growing up. The lack of physical exercise can be coupled with the availability of enormous amounts of highly processed food, often eaten in unsupervised environments.

If you are a parent with type 2 diabetes who wants to keep your children healthy, the best gift you can give them is to ensure that they are physically active and help them to eat right. There are many reasons to involve every member in a family with diabetes management, but when we look at the increase in type 2 in children, the concern should be translated into a high-volume wake-up call.

If your child has type 2, don't give up the fight. You can make a difference that will affect your child's entire future. Here are some things to do:

- Don't embarrass your child about his weight or eating habits in front of others—especially not his friends.
- Get information he can read on his own—the Internet is a great source.
- Get him moving. If it's difficult or embarrassing for him to be seen exercising with you, try hiring an older kid to get him to exercise.
- Work with him yourself. Often children are just manifesting the lifestyle issues of the entire family, which means that parents and other siblings need to be involved.

- Make your home a "health zone" by encouraging everyone who visits to live by the healthy rules you practice within.

In the past, pediatricians did not routinely test for type 2 in obese children. Now the increasing prevalence has brought greater awareness to the problem. In 1992, 2 to 4 percent of the cases of diabetes in children were type 2. By 1993 it rose to 16 percent. Recent studies show that the prevalence may be as high as 30 percent.

Eighty-five percent of all children diagnosed with type 2 are either overweight or obese. Seventy-four percent had a parent or immediate relative with type 2.
—*American Diabetes Association*

Ethnic Groups

There are a few ethnic groups for whom diabetes is almost an epidemic. Many families suffer from a number of instances of diabetes. But why does the disease occur more often in one race of people than another? Is it genetics that causes it or is it lifestyle? Well, as you may have guessed, with diabetes there are no easy answers. Let's take a look at the three groups that suffer the most from diabetes for more information.

African Americans

The incidence of diabetes among the African American population is almost twice as high as that for non-Hispanic whites. Here are the statistics: More than 2 million African Americans have diabetes and one half don't know it. Twenty-five percent of African Americans between the ages of 65 and 74 have diabetes, and one quarter of African American women over 55 have the disease. Diabetes is the fourth leading cause of death by disease in African Americans.

And once you have the disease as an African American man or

woman, statistically it is more likely that you'll suffer more from serious complications such as blindness, amputation, and kidney failure. Blindness due to diabetes is twice as high in African Americans than whites, and death rates are 27 percent higher than for whites with diabetes.

Why does diabetes have such a stranglehold on the African American population? Some researchers assign it to the "thrifty gene theory." Ancestors of current African Americans may have had a gene that allowed them to use food energy in an efficient manner so that during "feast or famine" cycles, survival would be maximized by slower rates of metabolism. In present-day America this genetic virtue has now become a possible cause for developing type 2 diabetes.

African American women are particularly plagued by type 2 diabetes. Among African Americans age 50 years or older, 19 percent of men and 28 percent of women have type 2 diabetes.
—*National Diabetes Information Clearinghouse/National Institutes of Health*

Another argument about why African Americans are so afflicted by diabetes is perhaps the cultural differences between African American and Caucasian women regarding size acceptance. In fact, for many, big is beautiful, and traditionally symbolizes prosperity and happiness in a woman. While this is a much healthier viewpoint psychologically than being obsessed with being skinny, physically it does open you up to more problems, especially the older and heavier you get.

Sheila, a 56-year-old African American, is a large woman. Obsessions about weight loss have never been a concern even when diagnosed with diabetes, she says, because her friends and neighbors (with or without diabetes) say, "Big is Beautiful." When this is accepted there is even less incentive to make the changes necessary to control blood sugar.

Food is such a pleasure and such a challenge in all ethnicities. Many of the wonderful flavors associated with the South and the African American community are not supportive of good diabetes control. But everyone wants to (and should be able to) enjoy food of their own ethnicity. Fabiola Gaines and Roniece Weaver concur: the authors of the recently released *The New Soul Food Cookbook for People with Diabetes* seek to make over traditional black recipes to make them healthier.

Hispanics

Hispanics have about the same chance of getting diabetes as African Americans, and with an expanding population, this makes diabetes a major issue for us all. Hispanics are two to four times more likely to have the disease than non-Hispanic whites, but less than half know they have it. Ten percent of all Mexican Americans have diabetes. Around a quarter of Mexican Americans and Puerto Rican Americans in the age group of 45 to 74 have diabetes. The rate for Cuban Americans is lower, but at 16 percent, is still relatively high.

The incidences of complications are much higher in this group. Mexican Americans are 4 to 6 percent more likely to have end-stage renal disease, although they do survive longer on dialysis than non-Hispanic whites. There is a higher incidence of retinopathy (twice the normal rate). Hispanic women have much higher complication and death rates during pregnancy than other women. But Hispanics are less likely to have a heart attack.

Why do Hispanics suffer so greatly from this disease? Part of the reason is genetics. If there has been an incidence of diabetes in your family, then you are more prone to get the disease as well. Also, many Hispanics have some Native American and African American lineage as well as Spanish, and as a result, they are more likely to inherit their higher rates of the disease.

There are also medical risk factors. Hispanics are more likely to suffer some of the precursors to diabetes, such as impaired glucose tolerance, insulin resistance, and gestational diabetes in women. Hispanics have a very high rate of obesity, with more Hispanic women getting the disease than men, and this may have something to do with the fact that their obesity levels are higher (nearly 50 percent of adult Mexican American women are overweight). And there is a great lack of physical exercise in the Hispanic population, with nearly 74 percent of Mexican American women reporting little or no leisure-time physical activity, and 65 percent of men reporting the same.

Many Hispanics delay treatment until serious complications have developed. This may have something to do with cultural and language barriers.

Native Americans

Diabetes is an epidemic for Native Americans. Of this population, 12.2 percent over the age of 19 has diabetes. In fact, one tribe in Arizona, the Pima tribe, has the highest rate of diabetes in the world. There, about 65 percent of the adults between the ages of 45 and 74 have diabetes.

Complications for Native Americans with diabetes are high. End-stage renal failure is six times more likely for this group, and amputations are 3 or 4 percent more likely for Native Americans.

Underserved Communities

Whatever the ethnicity, there are factors such as high-fat diets and overall poor nutrition that affect underserved communities. An unhealthy diet is oftentimes matched with a lack of exercise. For many who live in urban areas, there are myriad reasons why they don't get enough exercise. Everything that you need might be in your own neighborhood, thus causing you not to need to walk far for anything. The neighborhood may be too dangerous to go out and exercise after work. There may not be many parks in the area that are good for walks.

Many may not have access to good health care, either through lack of insurance or because there aren't many good doctors in the places where they live. It has also been argued that once diagnosed, the support systems are not in place for follow-up management and compliance. When priorities are centered on day-to-day survival, the long-term effects of diabetes are certainly put on the back burner.

I volunteer at a drug rehabilitation center on the Bowery in New York City. I met a man named Wayne who is 35 with type 2 diabetes. Wayne lives in a men's shelter and was asking me what he could do about his blurred vision and dizziness at certain times during the day. My first concern was his nutrition. The only breakfast available to him was highly sugared cereals or presweetened oatmeal. I felt foolish when I asked Wayne if he could get yogurt or cottage cheese, realizing that he could not. Finally, we figured his best strategy was to take the cheese sandwich snack available after dinner and use it for breakfast the next morning to make him feel less dizzy and keep his sugar under control throughout the day.

Outreach Programs

The American Diabetes Association sponsors a number of programs to help communities raise awareness about diabetes. This includes an outreach program to churches and synagogues called "Diabetes Sunday." At religious meetings, a guest speaker promotes screening for diabetes and is available to participants to answer questions. Another program is called "Get Up and Move." Its goal is to encourage exercise as part of an overall plan to control diabetes. These programs are focused on the African American community and targeted to those diagnosed or at a high risk for diabetes.

For the Native American community, so hard hit by diabetes, there is a program sponsored by the American Diabetes Association called "Awakening the Spirit" that reaches approximately 550 Native American communities with information about diabetes.

The Diabetes Assistance and Resources (DAR) program provides educational information for the Hispanic community. It promotes the importance of both prevention and control, and information is distributed in both English and Spanish. For more information on these programs, contact the American Diabetes Association.

———

As we examine different populations, stages in life, and gender, we can see individual differences in risk factors and complications in those with type 2 diabetes. But one message holds true no matter what group is observed: all of us need to be mindful of our lifestyle and the behaviors of our children in order to arrest the epidemic growth of diabetes. Any changes we can make affect our family, future generations, community, and country.

The key to making a difference is to take charge of the situation. Part 2 of this book lays out a life plan that should assist both groups and individuals to take life-altering and life-saving actions. Even small steps can make a difference.

part two

The Diabetes Life Plan

CHAPTER 4

Step-by-Step Plan for Weight Loss and Healthy Eating

I remember the day I decided I was fat. I was five years old and wearing a new dress. It was a sailor style, which was very popular in the 1950s: sleeveless with a big collar. I felt very special in this new dress and wanted to show my next-door neighbor. On my way over, I couldn't help but admire myself and the white piping on the collar, the crisp navy fabric, and the full skirt. As I looked down at the dress I caught sight of my shoulder near my armpit and something disrupted my view. I saw flesh. I saw fat! It bulged out of my dress and all around the armhole. From that moment on, it has been a daily battle. I don't think there has been a day in my life when I haven't thought about what I was eating and what size my body was.

Many of you may have similar stories. Whether you are 5 years old or 50, at some point the time comes to pay attention to your weight. Have you ever met anyone who doesn't want to lose weight? The thinnest, youngest, most beautiful women I know want to lose at least 5 pounds.

And then there are the rest of us! Most of us with type 2 diabetes have to lose at least some weight in order to control our blood sugar, because, as you read in chapter 1, being overweight contributes to developing diabetes and exacerbates conditions associated with complications. Weight loss can be beneficial to you by lowering cholesterol levels, blood pressure, triglycerides, and, of course, blood sugar levels.

The benefits rise as more weight loss occurs. There is a direct correlation between excess body weight and the resistance that cells have to insulin. Often, people can cease taking oral medications or they can cut down on their medications as weight loss progresses.

Whether you have some weight to lose or not, it is important for you to know that a healthy eating plan for those with diabetes is essentially the same as the way everyone else should eat in order to maintain a healthy lifestyle. You should not consider yourself burdened as a person with type 2 diabetes that you have to eat this way, because everyone should. It's just particularly important for you to be vigilant about eating healthy in order for you to be healthy.

Maybe you have tried many times to lose weight before, but now you *know* you have to do it for health reasons. There are many, many eating plans available, and perhaps you've already met with a nutritionist or diabetes educator and have created an individualized regimen, which is an important and useful course of action. Later in this chapter you'll find a review of several regimens. No matter what way of eating you choose, in the end it is all about the calories you consume. If you take in more calories than you burn every day, you will gain weight. If you take in fewer calories, you will lose weight. If you eat just 100 calories less a day than you burn, you'll be 10 pounds thinner in a year.

Essentially, weight loss can be reduced to one simple concept: You need to burn more calories than you take in. "Energy in, energy out." Consume fewer calories than you exert in exercise and daily activities and you will lose weight.

Those of us with diabetes need to be conscious of our food choices for the rest of our lives, so following a strict, highly regimented diet would feel like being in a straight jacket forever. Feeling so constrained, our natural reaction would be to break out of our shackles and let loose with a half-gallon of rocky road ice cream. That is why I'd like to propose a way of living rather than a "diet." This does include some "dos and don'ts," and you need to make some basic changes, which can be altered as you develop more control of your blood sugar. In addition, it allows you an avenue to travel when you find you have deviated out of control—a way for you to pull yourself back.

No one would ever consider me thin. I've never heard people say, "Eat a little more, you are too skinny." But now I fall into the normal range and this is one area of life where I am thrilled to be average. This wasn't a small accomplishment. Like many people, over the years I lost many pounds—over and over again. I went up and down with every diet available. None of them worked long term because I never looked at how I was going to eat for the rest of my life. I suppose as you get older the long view becomes a reality, as do the consequences of your actions. In a sense my attitude about eating changed with my diagnosis because I had to look at my lifestyle over time.

Sometimes when you set off to make changes, it's difficult to know just what to do first. If you follow the plan here step by step, it will allow you to develop a strategy that you can incorporate into your own lifestyle. That is what is so important—having a plan that fits into your particular lifestyle, which no one knows better than you.

When I was diagnosed and put myself on a new eating regimen, I was able to lose 37 pounds and keep it off. I did it by concentrating on one thing: my blood glucose levels. That's the system that I am sharing with you—a plan that uses your blood glucose levels as your primary guide. For example, if your readings are below 150 mg/dl, just above a normal range, you may be able to make some moderate adjustments in the way you eat now and be able to lose weight. If you do succeed in bringing it down, I've created a reward system for you. If you currently have higher blood sugar, I've given you some other important adjustments to make for your diet. Of course, consult your doctor or diabetes educator before you begin any new program.

For Those with Insulin Resistance

This plan will be quite effective if you have been told that your blood sugar levels are between 110 and 126 mg/dl. You are classified as insulin resistant, which means that you may be able to curtail full-fledged type 2 diabetes if you can lose some weight and get your blood sugar down to below 110.

According to Dr. Gerald Bernstein, former president of the American Diabetes Association, tight control through frequent monitoring is the best guide to control your blood sugar and your weight. See chapter 6 for further information on when to check your blood glucose levels.

But before we go further into my weight loss program, here is information you need to learn about what role food plays in your body. First let's look at what the different nutrients in our food are, and then we can look at how to put it all together into a plan that fits into your real life.

A Quick Lesson on Diabetes Nutrition

What Is Food "Made Of"?

You may have heard a lot about high-carbohydrate diets, high-protein diets, or low-fat diets. Every diet guru seems to be focusing on some element of a diet in order to show us how to lose weight. But what are carbohydrates, fats, and proteins, and why are they so important? Even if you don't have a pound to lose it's important to be an informed "consumer."

Let's examine the role of protein, fats, and carbohydrates in our diet.

The Role of Carbohydrates

Carbohydrates are a primary nutrient. They are critical for your nervous system and brain to function and are the prime source of energy for physical activity. This is the nutrient that contributes to most of our blood sugar and has the biggest effect on the rise and fall of glucose levels.

Carbohydrates are molecules of carbon, hydrogen, and water that are linked together. There are two kinds of carbohydrates—simple and complex—which we need to be mindful of. While they all eventually break down into glucose, some carbohydrates do it faster than others. Depending on how multiple the links are we either have simple carbohydrates, such as table sugar, or complex carbohydrates, such as whole grains. Because simple carbohydrates have a less complicated structure, they can be broken down and absorbed faster and go more quickly into your bloodstream, especially when eaten without fat or protein. Most of the foods we eat that have simple sugars also have fats or proteins with them; for example, ice cream has fat and protein. This slows the absorption rate of glucose, which is helpful to know but doesn't mean that these foods give us all the nutrients we require. On the other hand, complex carbohydrates can take longer to be digested and enter your bloodstream at a slower rate, especially since whole-grain products can also contain fiber. When carbohydrates are absorbed slowly, they will cause less spiking of your blood sugar.

When it comes to glucose control all carbohydrates are the same, but when it comes to nutrition and health there is a big difference. Carbohydrates are contained in bread, cereals, beans, legumes, dairy products, fruits, and vegetables. Cookies, cakes, and ice cream are also full of carbohydrates. It's up to each of us to decide where we want to "spend" our carbs on any given day.

Of course, carbohydrates are an essential part of any eating plan. They can be a quick source of energy and some have lots of important vitamins, minerals, and fiber in them. However, if excess amounts of carbohydrates are being consumed—more than your body can use—they are stored as glycogen in the liver and muscles. Later, glycogen can be burned off for energy. After that, any carbohydrate excess is converted to fat and then stored (usually in all the wrong places). That's why it's important to control the amount of carbohydrates we consume. It doesn't just raise your blood sugar, it creates fat. And that fat, especially when you are over 40, tends to settle in your middle. Why is this particularly dangerous? This is the fat that researchers find contributes most to heart disease, because it is so close to your most vital organs. By cutting out simple sugars we cut out extra calories, with few nutrients, and we cut out foods that quickly raise our glucose level.

For most adults, 45 to 75 grams of carbohydrates per meal is sufficient depending on age, weight, and physical activity. This translates into three to five servings each meal every day. For good health, your carbohydrates should be spread out between whole grains, fruits and vegetables, and dairy products.

Glycemic Effect of Food

There are other considerations regarding how quickly carbohydrates are converted to glucose in your bloodstream. It's called the glycemic effect of food. There has been a great deal of scientific research about how certain carbohydrates raise or lower our blood sugar at different rates. Tests have been performed by administering certain foods and then observing how fast the blood sugar rises in a measured amount of time. Some of the results are quite surprising. For example, pretzels seem to affect the blood sugar faster than peanuts. White potatoes have a higher glycemic effect than sweet potatoes. Foods with a low glycemic effect produce a slow, steady glucose level. While this information may be useful to many people, it is particularly important to those of us with any sort of insulin resistance. Because we are extremely sensitive to the rise and fall of blood sugar, it's a good idea to choose as many foods as possible from the low or medium list or at least balance the high-glycemic foods with low ones.

Here is a list of some common foods and their glycemic effect. For further information consult *The Glucose Revolution* by Jennie Brand-Miller et al.

High-Glycemic Foods
Cornflakes
Pretzels
Rice cakes
Bagels
Corn chips
Watermelon

Medium-Glycemic Foods
White rice
Brown rice
Bananas
Popcorn
Cantaloupe

Low-Glycemic Foods
Oatmeal
Bulgur wheat
Oranges
Tomato soup
Yogurt
Skim milk
Lentils
Grapefruit
Soybeans

Starch and Fiber
Starch and fiber are carbohydrates. Starch is the storage form of carbohydrates for plants. As plants grow, they store energy for future use. So when we eat potatoes, grains, and seeds, we are consuming that concentrated energy. And energy is another term for calories.

Fiber is the supportive part of plants, such as stems, leaves, and seeds. Not all of it is broken down when we eat it, but it provides many benefits by aiding in digestion and slowing down the time it takes for food to pass through our digestive tract. This allows for a feeling of fullness and satiety. It causes absorption to occur at a slower rate as food is broken down, which means that we don't have such a quick rise in our blood sugar.

There are two types of fiber: insoluble and soluble. Insoluble fiber can help reduce constipation and may aid in the risk reduction of colon and other cancers. Research has shown that it also helps reduce blood glucose levels. Examples of insoluble fiber are whole-grain products, wheat bran, beans, and many fruits and vegetables. Soluble fiber can reduce cholesterol levels by attaching to the cholesterol in the intestines and then removing it from the body. It can also lower glucose levels by slowing the rate of digestion and absorption of carbohydrates. Beans have soluble fiber. Other sources are oat bran, barley, oatmeal, and psyllium husk.

You should have 20 to 35 grams of fiber in your diet per day; however, consider a gradual increase of fiber to avoid uncomfortable bloating, cramping, and gas. Look at this list and see how you could add more fiber to your diet.

Fiber in Foods

Brown rice, ½ cup 1 g	Lentils, ½ cup 3.7 g
Carrots, ½ cup cooked 3 g	Green peas, ½ cup 3.6 g
Corn, ½ cup 2.9 g	Apple, medium 3.5 g
Kidney beans, ½ cup 7.3 g	Pear, 1 large 3.1 g
Navy beans, ½ cup 6 g	Prunes, 3 3 g
Dried figs, 2 4 g	Raspberries, 1 cup 8.4 g
Bran flakes, ¾ cup 4 g	Air-popped popcorn, 1 cup 1 g
Raisin bran, ¾ cup 4 g	Wheat germ, ¼ cup 3.4 g
Whole-wheat spaghetti, 1 cup 3.9 g	Whole-wheat bread, 1 slice 1 g

A Note about Whole Wheat

You may see a product that is labeled as whole wheat. Check the ingredients carefully. Often whole wheat is included in very small quantities and the product, like some kinds of whole-wheat bread, has more white flour than any other ingredient.

The Role of Protein

If carbohydrates provide the fuel for your body, then protein provides much of the support we need to build muscles, connective tissue, and cell structures. We can find protein in meat, fish, chicken, eggs, some dairy products, as well as legumes, seeds, and soy products.

Proteins are comprised of a series of molecular structures called amino acids. Similar to carbohydrates, when we eat proteins they are broken down into smaller units, amino acids, and absorbed by the cells.

Some of these amino acids are essential: we need to get them from food we eat and don't produce them in the body. That's why it's important that we have sufficient protein in our diet. Since the body is constantly rebuilding and remodeling cells using protein, we must replenish protein every day. If the body doesn't get protein through diet, it will break down tissue in order to release amino acids necessary to rebuild other tissues and cells. This will eventually leave us weak and depleted. Yet most people in the United States usually have an abundance of protein in the diet. About 10 to 20 percent of our total daily calories should come from protein. It's very easy to consume this amount, as it equals only 6 to 8 ounces per day. Think about the size of a deck of cards or the palm of a woman's hand, and that's roughly the 3-ounce serving size of protein for lunch and dinner.

We want to consume the best quality protein possible to provide all the amino acids we need with the lowest amounts of fat. That's why if we eat red meat, we should only eat a minimum amount, choosing the leanest cuts and trimming excess fat. When we eat poultry, a good source of protein, we should remove the skin and eat the white meat.

There are several popular diets promoting large intakes of protein, including the Atkins Diet. This is quite taxing on the filtering system of your kidneys, which is of particular concern to those with diabetes. Kidneys are already strained as diabetes progresses. See "Complications" in chapter 2 for more information on kidney disease in those with diabetes.

The Role of Fat

Although we need to be mindful of the type and quantity of fat we consume, we do require it in our diet. We need dietary fat to insulate and protect our internal organs, transport certain vitamins—such as A, D, E, and K—throughout the body, and give us a sense of satiety (fullness). Fat is so energy dense that 1 gram provides more than twice the calories that carbohydrates or proteins provide. This may have been very useful to cavemen as they fought the saber-toothed tiger, and it still can be useful to highly active people, but for most of us, excess dietary fat can affect our hearts, waistline, and even blood sugar.

The other big issue with the consumption of fat is the type of fat we consume. Saturated fat is a buzzword you might be hearing a lot about in commercials. What's the difference? These are the types of fats we normally find in food:

■ Saturated: This is fat that is dense and remains solid at room temperature, such as butter, lard, and shortening, as well as palm oil, animal products, and high-fat cheese. Saturated fat not only is dense when we look at the package, it remains thick when consumed and coats our arteries and veins, contributing to heart disease.

■ Unsaturated: An unsaturated fat is usually liquid at room temperature, like oils. There are two types of unsaturated fat: monounsaturated and polyunsaturated. Polyunsaturated fat is mainly found in safflower, cottonseed, and soybean oils. Monounsaturated fats include olive and canola oil and may help lower your blood cholesterol levels and help your body fight against heart disease.

■ Trans fatty acids: When unsaturated fats are hydrogenated, they become what is known as trans fatty acids. Hydrogenation is a process in which food technologists are able to convert a liquid unsaturated fat into a more densely, easily spread fat such as margarine. You can also find partially hydrogenated fats in processed foods and certain oils. An excess of trans fatty acids is thought to contribute to certain cancers and heart disease.

■ Cholesterol: This is a waxy fat substance found in animal products. When eaten in excess, animal products, which contain saturated fat, can raise our blood cholesterol levels. It is also made in the liver and used by the body to make certain hormones and cell structures.

Of the calories we consume every day we can have about 30 percent from fat, but only 10 percent or less of our daily calories should be from saturated fat, with the remaining 20 percent from unsaturated sources. That means that if you eat 2,000 calories a day, you should have less than 65 grams of total fat, which should include no more than 20 grams of saturated fat. A teaspoon of oil is equal to 5 grams or 45 calories. Just because certain fats, such as monounsaturates, are better for us than hydrogenated fats, contained in most margarine, it doesn't mean that we should be swimming in olive oil. Portion control is still required. (We'll discuss more about portion control later in the chapter.)

With this information in hand, we are ready to begin our basic plan. This is the method that I used to lose weight and keep it off.

Carol Guber's Eating Plan

STEP ONE: PREPARATION

1. Buy the following items. Each will be used in this plan.

A digital scale on which to weigh yourself
A full-length mirror
Measuring cups

Measuring spoons
A kitchen scale

2. *Weigh yourself once a week and write it down.*

Your mind will do strange things with the numbers on the scale. Don't rely on your memory. It's best to weigh yourself at the same time each week, preferably in the morning without clothes on. Keep records so you won't forget where you have been and where you are going. As you progress, you can feel very good about how far you've come.

3. *Look at yourself in a full-length mirror without clothes on at least once a day.*

This can be a new, and sometimes painful, chore for some of us, but it will help keep you on track and you'll see if you've made any progress with your weight loss. Too many of us just look at mirrors that show us from the waist up. We do this even when dressed. This does not give us the full impact of our weight gain or loss.

Your daily visit with the mirror will provide you with an opportunity to appreciate your body all over again. Get to know it—it's a hard-working machine—and you will celebrate more in its changing shape as you lose weight.

4. *Practice measuring food.*

Portion control is the biggest issue in losing weight. Many of us are aware of what kinds of foods we should eat, but the amount we eat leaves much to chance and spur-of-the moment decisions. It's important to measure, but don't wait until you are going to eat it. Who wants to bring measuring cups to the dinner table? Who wants to stand in the kitchen with a scale when your family is waiting for you? Learn proper measurements when you can be objective. Put the food on a dinner plate to give you perspective.

Take some time when you are relaxed and not hungry. I've listed some common foods to measure. You probably have your own favorites. Perhaps you want to do this with other members of your family or friends, so that you can all learn what proper portions should look like. Throughout the chapter we will discuss what constitutes a proper portion. In addition, refer to the American Diabetes Association Exchange Lists for Meal Planning.

Use your measuring cups, spoons, and scale to measure some portions of foods you enjoy eating. Pick some from the list below. The menus in the back of the book will give you an indication of the portions that are appropriate for a healthy life plan. How big is an appropriate portion of boneless chicken breast? It is about 3 to 4 ounces. Do you like hamburgers? Take out a scale and see how much you think is "normal," and compare that with a portion size that most nutritionists think is the right size (about 3 ounces, equaling 225 calories).

As you look at appropriate portions, remember that you want to spread your nutrients throughout the day, especially your carbohydrates. However, if you end up with more at one meal, try cutting back at the next.

Starch/Cereals/Grains (approximately 80 calories, 15 grams carbohydrate)

Bread, 1 slice (1 oz)

Hot dog or hamburger bun, ½

Roll, 1 small plain (1 oz)

Cereals, unsweetened, ½ cup

Grape-Nuts, ¼ cup

Oats, ½ cup

Pasta, ½ cup

Rice, ⅓ cup

Beans, ½ cup

Peas, ½ cup

Corn, ½ cup

Potato, baked, 3 oz

Graham crackers, 3 squares

Melba toast, 4

Popcorn (low-fat microwave or popped with no fat), 3 cups

Milk (approximately 90 calories, 12 grams carbohydrate)

Skim or 1%, 1 cup

Low-fat buttermilk, 1 cup

Nonfat plain yogurt, ¾ cup

Fruit (approximately 60 calories, 15 grams carbohydrate)

Apple, small, 1 (4 oz)

Banana, medium, ½

Cantaloupe, small, ⅓ melon (11 oz) or 1 cup cubes

Orange, small, 1

Peach, medium, 1 (6 oz)

Pineapple, fresh, ¾ cup

Raisins, 2 tablespoons

Orange juice, ½ cup

Apple juice, ½ cup

Vegetables (approximately 25 calories, 5 grams carbohydrate)

Most vegetables, ½ cup

Except for starchy vegetables like peas, carrots, and potatoes, consider them unlimited. Most people have more difficulty eating 2 to 5 vegetables per day rather than ever limiting them.

Meat and Meat Substitute (approximately 55–75 calories per ounce, no carbohydrate). Remember: A portion of meat is usually 3–4 ounces.

Chicken or turkey, 1 oz

Veal cutlet, 1 oz

Tuna, canned in water, 1 oz

Shellfish, 1 oz

Feta cheese, 1 oz

Cottage cheese, ¼ cup

Grated Parmesan cheese, 2 tablespoons

Whole egg, 1

Egg whites, 2

Tofu, ½ cup

Fats (approximately 45 calories)
Oil, 1 teaspoon
Peanut butter, 2 teaspoons
Cream cheese, 1 tablespoon
Mayonnaise, 1 teaspoon
Mayonnaise (reduced fat), 1 tablespoon
Butter, 1 teaspoon

Take a good look—is it the size of a fist, your thumb? Try to get a visual image to refer to in the future of what a good portion should look like.

Portion control is an essential component in healthy eating. How to visualize a portion? Here are a few everyday objects that you can use to approximate a portion:

A serving of pasta = tennis ball
A baked potato = computer mouse
A serving of cheese = set of dice
A serving of protein = deck of cards

Step Two: Follow a Simple Plan

The plan is based on several basic principles, which are described in detail in the following section.

1. Base your eating plan on your glucose level.
2. Higher glucose levels require tighter control, while lower levels allow for more liberty. These are called Levels 1, 2, and 3 in this book.

This plan will produce results because it has the essential elements to continue eating right for a lifetime: variety, moderation, and balance.

■ *Variety:* This diet offers us many different types of food to maintain our interest.

■ *Moderation:* Our meals should include portion control.

■ *Balance:* We want to make sure that we are consuming sufficient water, vitamins, minerals, proteins, and carbohydrates while limiting fat consumption.

Eat breakfast, lunch, and dinner and two snacks per day.

 A Note about the "Quick Fix"

For many of us, the resolve to alter our eating takes a great deal of inner strength. It also may have taken a great deal of courage to face how we got into this situation in the first place. Where did those extra pounds come from? It would be nice to receive an instant reward just for making the decision to lose weight—5 pounds off for determination and 10 for starting a new plan. Unfortunately, it doesn't happen that way. Any program that promotes on Tuesday that you'll be able to lose weight by Saturday night is bogus.

Remember, any worthwhile weight loss plan takes time. Stay on this plan for six weeks and you will see a difference. Quick plans that promise fast results cannot be sustained over time. And with diabetes it's important to look at the long haul, as this is a disease you need to be able to control for the rest of your life. No quick fixes, no instant cures. Many nutritionists feel that the best diet for diabetes control is the same as a normal, healthy diet that even people without diabetes should be following. We are promoting good, nutritious food coupled with a sensible physical activity plan. The goal is to lose weight and control diabetes with diet and exercise alone for as long as you possibly can.

This is a plan based on how high your blood sugar level is when you begin a weight loss program. Very often if you can reduce your blood sugar levels, your weight, cholesterol, and blood pressure will also be reduced.

As we have discussed, in order to lose weight we must somehow eat fewer calories than we burn on any given day. It's also essential that we get the highest quality nutrients from the calories we consume. When we eat a lot of sugar and fat we are eating "empty calories," calories that don't provide important vitamins, minerals, or protein and other building blocks for our body. And excess sugar in itself can boost our triglycerides, dangerous fats in our blood that can lead to heart disease. In addition, for those of us with type 2 diabetes, we must consider the effect our food intake has on our blood glucose levels.

The other element in this plan is to cut out white flour, which provides little fiber and much fewer valuable nutrients than whole grains do. For instance, it would be much more beneficial for you to substitute a serving of pasta made with white flour with a serving of beans, which provides lots of fiber and is rich in protein.

Level 1: Recently Diagnosed and Glucose Levels of 126–150 mg/dl

If your glucose level is only moderately high, you may be able to continue eating mostly as you do but eliminate or radically cut back on added sugar and white flour, using the Food Guide Pyramid as a general guide. This method is especially useful if you don't have a great deal of weight to lose. This plan concentrates on lowering the consumption of foods that could raise your glucose level. Keep an eye on the Food Guide Pyramid for additional guidelines. Developed from research by the United States Department of Agriculture, the pyramid outlines what to eat each day in a fashion that allows you to adapt it to individual needs. That's why it is referred to as a guide, not a set of rules.

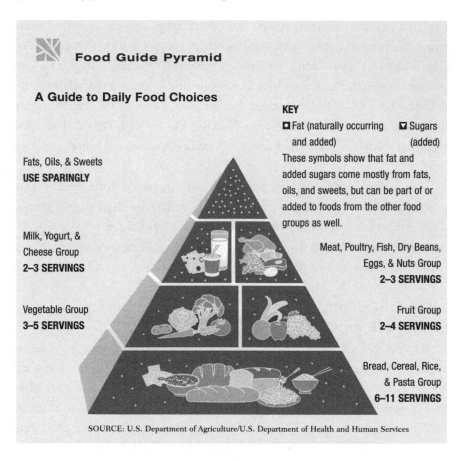

Food Guide Pyramid

A Guide to Daily Food Choices

KEY
■ Fat (naturally occurring   ☑ Sugars
   and added)   (added)
These symbols show that fat and added sugars come mostly from fats, oils, and sweets, but can be part of or added to foods from the other food groups as well.

Fats, Oils, & Sweets
USE SPARINGLY

Milk, Yogurt, &
Cheese Group
2–3 SERVINGS

Meat, Poultry, Fish, Dry Beans,
Eggs, & Nuts Group
2–3 SERVINGS

Vegetable Group
3–5 SERVINGS

Fruit Group
2–4 SERVINGS

Bread, Cereal, Rice,
& Pasta Group
6–11 SERVINGS

SOURCE: U.S. Department of Agriculture/U.S. Department of Health and Human Services

It sounds fairly straightforward. Here we are looking at processed foods, condiments, baked goods, and many convenience foods. Beware of processed foods, especially those labeled "low fat." Often low-fat products replaced some of the flavor with higher amounts of sugar. When you become more aware of sugar in food you'll see that it lurks in many foods and in many forms. Be vigilant when you read a food label. Ingredients are listed starting with the largest amount first. When reading labels, check for any of the following sugars:

Beet sugar
Brown sugar
Cane sugar

Confectioner's sugar
Cornstarch
Corn sweetener
Corn syrup
Dextrose
Fructose
Granulated sugar
Honey
Invert sugar
Lactose
Levulose
Maltose
Maple syrup
Molasses
Raw syrup
Sorghum
Sucrose
Sugar cane syrup

Also be on the lookout for:

■ Sugar alcohols
These are sweeteners that are often used in foods listed as "contains no sugar." However, they can be high in calories—2 to 3 calories per gram as compared with sugar at 4 calories per gram. They can also be hard on the digestion for some people, causing upset stomachs and diarrhea. Examples of this sugar are sorbitol and mannitol.

■ Sugar substitutes
We commonly see three different artificial sweeteners: aspartame (Equal), saccharin (Sweet'n Low), and acesulfame K. Many doctors and dietitians allow for moderate amounts of these sugars in your diet; however, there are other factors to be considered. Don't think that artificial sweeteners will help you lose weight. A "diet" drink with a pizza is not going to take off calories. There are also scientific studies suggesting that people who consume large quantities of artificial

sweeteners tend to also consume large quantities of carbohydrates. In fact, according to Lewis Mehl-Madrona, M.D., at Beth Israel Hospital New York, they may even promote carbohydrate cravings.

Breaking the Sweet-Tooth Habit

If you are someone who is obsessed with sugary foods, it may be best to cut them entirely out of your diet until you can control yourself and only have a treat once in a while. For some people, just being told they can't have sugar can create a craving.

S.F., a successful businessman, was 55 years old when diagnosed with diabetes. Before then, he rarely had dessert and never ate chocolate. Gradually, he became obsessed with sweets and even ate chocolate bars when alone. The thought of being denied something increased his desire. He had to gather the support of his family and even his employees to keep him from eating chocolate and desserts. He reports that it took three weeks of staying away from chocolate to stop eating it as a habit. It takes daily vigilance to maintain his resolve, but now that he is in good control, a sweet from time to time can be incorporated into his overall food plan.

You can break the sweet tooth habit. Eating three meals a day on time helps, because fluctuating glucose levels can aggravate your craving. It also helps to have a buddy or loved one who is attempting to break the habit too. A small amount of sugar is okay as long as it fits into an overall daily plan. If you have had several servings of bread at each meal, cereal, potatoes, rice (all carbohydrates), it may not be a good day to have cake for dessert after dinner. On the other hand, if you anticipate a special night out, skip the breadbasket, watch your fat intake, and have a moderate treat.

A Note about Checking Labels

Here's a rule of thumb when reading a food label: If there are 5 grams or less of sugar per serving you have a green light to eat it. More than that means that the food is a treat and you should limit it.

About White Flour

Substitute whole-grain flour for white flour wherever you can. Whole grains tend to offer more nutrients per serving and tend to have more fiber. Remember, you want to get as many nutrients as possible for your calories. Whole-grain foods have more fiber and vitamins and minerals. Again, this is an issue of glucose control combined with health. One reason I recommend cutting down on white flour is because it is so easy to identify it as a carbohydrate.

There is another pitfall of white flour. It tends to be the main ingredient in foods that come in gigantic sizes. Now we see bagels, muffins, and rolls the size of bowling balls—and the portion size keeps growing. According to Lisa Young, Ph.D., expert in portion control, the average bagel is three to five times the size it used to be, and what the Food Guide Pyramid recommends. The Food Guide Pyramid suggests one half of a bagel, equaling 90 calories, as a serving. But when we think we are being reasonable by eating half a bagel, we are probably eating five times the amount we should. Today the average bagel is 550 calories, according to Dr. Young. Again, this is a sign that "supersize" portions need to be avoided!

If we watch our white flour consumption we will automatically eliminate extra calories and often extra carbohydrates.

Try this plan for six weeks and see if your blood sugar goes down. For some, this will work well, especially if you combine it with additional exercise (see chapter 5). I have found that people who are recently diagnosed and have a reasonable yet slightly indulgent eating pattern can pull themselves together with this simple approach. If you do see results and you can keep or sustain a blood glucose level of 125 mg/dl for the six weeks thereafter without medication, then you could have a treat—such as a dessert or a big bagel—once a week.

Each of us has been diagnosed at different stages in diabetes. For those who have blood sugar above 150 mg/dl and cannot bring it down by cutting out sugar and white flour, move on to the next level.

Level 2: Glucose Levels of 150–200 mg/dl

While following the advice for the Level 1 plan by continuing to eliminate sugar and white flour, make adjustments to the following:

Fruit

Make sure you have two pieces of fruit per day. If you are having more than that, cut it down to just two. Fruit contains a sugar called fructose, which is metabolized differently than other simple sugars. Fruits are so rich in vitamins and fiber that we shouldn't be without them. What does it mean when we say two pieces? This is where portion control and scales are important. Follow the guideline below for fruit size and weight. If you have your choice, it's better to have fewer tropical fruits such as bananas, mangoes, and pineapple. These tend to raise your blood sugar faster than other fruits, which have a lower glycemic effect. Also, fruit eaten with a little bit of protein will slow the rise in blood sugar. Try having an apple with a tablespoon of peanut butter or grapes with an ounce of low-fat cheese.

Eat two servings daily of

- Small apple or orange, or
- ½ banana, or
- 1 cup of fresh berries or melon, or
- Grapes (15)

Note: Avoid fruit juices. They make your blood sugar rise too quickly.

Dairy

Eat two servings of

- 1 cup of nonfat or low-fat milk, or
- 1 cup of nonfat or low-fat yogurt, or
- 1 cup of buttermilk

Note: Consider higher-fat cheese more as fat and protein rather than part of the dairy category alone. That includes cottage cheese.

Fiber

Raise your fiber by increasing your consumption of beans, whole grains, and vegetables. You should have 20 to 35 grams of fiber a day. If you are new to eating so much fiber, start slowly. You may have quite a bit of gas in the beginning. Refer back to the list earlier in the chapter and remember that there are many ways of incorporating fiber, from beans in your salad to more nonstarchy vegetables to lots of whole grains.

Eat three meals a day and two snacks and make sure you eat breakfast. It's so important that you maintain even blood sugar levels. When you don't have breakfast you are trying to function on depleted stores of glucose. Your levels can go way down. Then when you do eat it will force your levels up at a fast pace.

Ideally, you can follow this plan and have your blood sugar in control without the need of oral medications. In the process, you should be able to lose weight and keep it off. It's difficult to predict how much weight you can lose, because so much depends on your own metabolism and activity level. But if you can maintain this plan and stay in control you will notice that your weight will begin to shift.

Level 3: Glucose Levels Over 200 mg/dl

If your blood sugar is above 200 mg/dl, you need to begin with a more organized plan. The result will be weight loss, a drop in blood sugar, and in many cases the elimination of oral medication or a decrease in the amount.

Exchange System: American Diabetes Association Plan

This is a dietary planning system that organizes food into categories or "exchanges." In each category, all the serving sizes are considered equal in the amount of calories, protein, carbohydrates, and fats. This offers flexibility and variety since one exchange can be substituted for another in the same category. For example, in the plan you could have one slice of bread or ⅓ cup of rice—they are equal. For further information, refer to the American Diabetes Association Exchange Lists for Meal Planning. This should be planned with a nutritionist or certified diabetes educator.

A Note about "Exchanges," Portions, and Servings

Sometimes people can be confused by terms like portions or servings or exchanges. In the exchange system, foods are listed together because they have similar nutritive value, including calories. You can have more than one exchange from a list for any meal. In fact, you may want to have several at a time. For example, an exchange of meat is 1 ounce, but you would have 3 to 4 ounces to equal a full portion. An exchange of rice is ½ cup, but you could have a 1-cup portion and include that as two exchanges. See the chart below, which indicates the number of exchanges per meal you should consume according to the number of calories you consume per day. See page 67 for a list of everyday foods with calories and exchange sizes.

Exchange	1,200 calories	1,500 calories	1,800 calories	2,000 calories	2,200 calories
Starch	6	7	8	9	11
Meat	4	5	6	6	6
Vegetable	3	4	5	5	5
Fruit	2	2	2	3	3
Milk (nonfat)	2	2	2	3	3
Fat	3	5	6	7	8

Summary of Carol Guber's Step-by-Step Plan

Level	Glucose	Eat
1	126–150 mg/dl	Eliminate/cut down on table sugar, white flour.
2	150 mg/dl–200 mg/dl	Have no more or less than 2 servings of fruit per day. No more than 2 servings of dairy per day. Slowly increase fiber to 20 to 30 grams per day.
3	Over 200 mg/dl	Follow the ADA exchange system.

Other Diets

The plan and tips that I have set out represent a simple, direct approach. However, you may want to follow some other system. If so, there are some questions you should ask yourself. How do you choose a weight loss plan? What does that mean in practical terms? How do I decide what diet to use? Here is a review of several kinds of diets. Which one will make you feel the happiest? Which one will be the easiest for you to follow and understand?

In practical terms, look for diets that

- You can sustain for a lifetime
- Support eating as a social and family activity
- Are easy to follow—involve only a simple plan
- You know what you should and shouldn't eat with a quick glance at a plate
- Can honor your own ethnicity

The United States may be a melting pot, but we should be able to have unique foods that reflect our own cultural roots. If we search back into our roots, we can find nourishing foods that are true to our heritage. We should be able to enjoy these foods and incorporate them into an eating plan. What is your heritage? Look back a hundred years and find foods associated with your background.

Avoid diets that

- Severely limit or excessively promote one kind of food (where you lose weight if you eat only pineapples and pizza)
- Propose you eat excessive amounts of only one category of food such as high carbohydrate or high protein
- Force you to be tied to exact measurements (You don't want to carry a scale and measuring cups everywhere you go!)
- Force you to special-order high-priced food only

Below is a list of some weight loss plans. Of course, check with your doctor, nutritionist, or diabetes educator before you begin.

Carbohydrate Counting

This is a method of counting only the carbohydrates you consume each day, which has several benefits. If you need to lose weight it helps in calculating your daily calorie intake by controlling the amount of carbs you eat. It will also assist you in spreading your carbs throughout the day so that you'll keep your blood sugar on a more even keel.

The basis of carb counting is that most servings of carbs are 15 grams, which equals about 90 calories. The foods that contain carbs are fruits, vegetables, milk, meat, sugar, and candies. Protein and fat don't contain carbs, so they aren't counted. This may be a pitfall of this system, since you could be eating an appropriate amount of carbohydrates but still consuming too much fat and gain weight. You can count by using the exchange list; figure that one exchange of fruit, milk, starch, or three exchanges of vegetables equals 15 grams (that's about 60 to 80 calories). It's best to try to eat the same number of carbs every day and about the same amount at each meal. People with type 1 diabetes often count carbs to determine the amount of insulin to use.

Weight Watchers

A highly effective program based on a system of points for food and activity. The program allows for points to be customized based on individual preferences. The group meetings offer support, camaraderie, and a sense of control. Weight Watchers group leaders all have successfully completed the program themselves. There is now an online program available on the organization's website, www.weightwatch-ers.com.

High-Protein Diets

There are several high-protein diets, including the Atkins Diet, that are very popular because people can experience fast results of weight loss in a short amount of time. These diets allow you to eat large amounts of protein, including large amounts of bacon and cheese. However, there are many long-term problems with these diets:

- It's hard to maintain the weight loss in the long run. If you go off the diet, you'll gain back the weight lost.
- There is a lack of fiber in the diet.
- There are too few vegetables and fruit, so that valuable nutrients are missing.
- There can be excessive amounts of saturated fat, which can contribute to heart disease.

Glycemic Index

The glycemic index is based on research that has found different carbohydrates produce different effects on the blood glucose level because of their rates of digestion. All carbohydrates are rated on a scale of 1 to 100. Carbohydrates are grouped as low-, medium-, or high-glycemic foods. Some are listed on page 61. There is some debate regarding judging a food individually without the other foods it is consumed with. In addition, some think that we all have different reactions to carbohydrates within our own bodies, and we may not all react the same.

Food Diaries

You may be asked by your nutritionist or diabetes educator to keep a food diary for a limited period of time, usually three days to a week. That will allow you to look at your food consumption and eating patterns in a way that can allow counseling and changes. Sometimes it can be daunting to look at this straight on, but it will ultimately assist you in your goals.

Step Three: Set Up Some Rules for Eating

 Don't eat anything you can't lift.   —Miss Piggy

I couldn't be in the position to control my eating if I hadn't taken the time to figure out what triggers my snacking. So I do my best to keep a few rules about eating. I use these with my clients. See if they work for you. Perhaps you have some similar ones or you can develop ones that work for you.

- If you can't control it, cut it out.

Although no food should be taboo, I recommend that if you can't control eating a certain food, cut it out of your diet altogether—at least until you can moderate your craving. For example, I have a client who is obsessed with cheese. Once she starts eating she can't discriminate between a 1-ounce square of cheddar or half a wheel. She just keeps going and adds tons of crackers for good measure. So the best decision was to cut all cheese from her diet. Because she eliminated this completely, she developed a quick reaction whenever she is asked, "Would you like some cheese?" Her reply is now: "Oh no, I never eat it." Of course, if she could control the amount of cheese when offered it would be a perfectly acceptable food. Look at food that seems to cause you to react this way. A certain sweet? Bread? Do these trigger a response that causes you to keep eating?

- Don't skip meals—stay on a schedule.

You need to keep your blood sugar steady. When you skip a meal, your blood sugar can go down and you could end up overeating at the next meal or making poor choices later in the day. Also, these highs and lows cause greater insulin resistance. Staying on schedule will help you feel more in control about food issues and your body will respond. Sometimes skipping meals is a sign that you are not allowing your well-being to be the priority it should.

- Don't let yourself feel too hungry.

We all make poor eating decisions when we're hungry. Think about hunger on a scale of 1 to 5—5 being completely full and 1 being as starving as if you were stranded on a desert island. It's best to try to maintain a level 3 most of the day. Don't eat when you are a 5 or even 4, and don't let yourself get down to a 1. When we let ourselves get too hungry, we end up making decisions that aren't necessarily the most wise or positive for our health. But don't use this tip as a way of munching all day! A day-long buffet of snacking will throw off the best of eating plans. You can't judge how much you are actually eating if you are snacking all day. And even an additional extra 100 calories a day will add up to 10 pounds in a year.

- Slow down and enjoy your food.

Since eating is such a pleasure, why rush it? Savor it and you'll enjoy it even more. Eating is one of the great joys of life, not a race to the finish line. Besides, the faster we eat, the more we are going to want. It takes time for your stomach to signal your brain that it is full. Think about quality not quantity. When eating, try to think about chewing your food slowly, don't gobble and swallow. The more times you chew each mouthful, the easier your food is to digest and the longer it will take you to eat. This means that you can get more pleasure out of less food. Try putting your knife and fork down occasionally while eating. It will help slow things down a bit.

- Don't eat if you are upset.

I tend to eat more when I am upset, but end up enjoying the food less. So it just isn't worth the calories to continue to eat when aggravated. If I find myself upset while I am eating, I try to stop while I am in that state. I just put my fork down and breathe a little. If I keep eating when agitated, it's hard for me to even realize how much I've consumed or even that I've been munching at all. Then I'll look at my plate and think, "Where did all the food go?" Of course, it isn't always possible to follow this tip, but even if you can stop for just a minute, you'll benefit greatly.

■ No second helpings.

The first plate of food is not what puts on weight, it's the second and third. Give up that whole idea of seconds. Place the amount of food on your plate that is appropriate and that is all you should have. When I work with my private clients or members of my support group at NYU, I've noticed that people learn fairly fast about portion size. That's not the problem. Remember that you should practice weighing your food so by the time a meal comes around you have a good sense of what a portion consists of.

One client enjoyed spending long amounts of time at the dinner table. This is where friends and family gathered, shared stories, and were in contact at the end of the day. The longer she sat, however enjoyable that might be, the more she would eat. Second helpings were followed by . . . picking. She didn't want to leave the table because that's where the fun was, so we created a signal to stop eating. First she would fill her plate only once with the proper amount of food. After she was finished, she took a bit of hand cream and applied it to her hands. This was a signal to herself that eating was over, and now she has the smoothest hands on the Upper East Side. The scent of hand cream also helped to displace the lingering food smell too! Some people have success when they brush their teeth right away or have a breath mint. When I am determined to eat, this has never stopped me. However, as a signal that the party is over, it may be useful.

- Don't snack while watching TV.

There is something about the food-TV connection that can be tough on even the strongest resolve. Television is mesmerizing on its own, and that hypnotic feeling can lead you down the wicked path of uncontrolled snacking. It can make you walk in a daze right into the kitchen for that extra-large treat. Don't get out the treats while watching TV. If you are hungry, eat at your kitchen table, away from the commercials for pizza and chips!

- There's no such thing as "going off the wagon."

If you eat something that doesn't really fit into the plan you've made for yourself, put down the whip and stop beating yourself up. One piece of cake is not going to be the deciding factor in your overall plan. What does count is not using that as an excuse to start putting the entire refrigerator into your mouth. So don't use this information as a way to rationalize eating food that you could just as easily pass up with a little discipline, and don't use the incident as another way of feeling bad. Just get on with it.

- You have to use up more calories than you consume in order to lose weight.

You can accomplish this by eating less, moving more, or covering all bases by doing both. Although you may be able to initially lose some weight without much exercise, it is almost impossible to maintain weight loss without increasing your physical activity as part of a lifetime strategy. Exercise will help shift your metabolism, create more muscle mass, lower your blood sugar, and help develop stronger bones for a lifetime. Just as important, it will help curb your appetite and give you a sense of well-being. See chapter 5 for inspiration and advice.

Step Four: Look Inside Yourself

If losing weight were so simple, we would just need to pick any popular diet book off the bookstore shelves, follow the instructions, and behold: you're a dream size 8 or a perfect 44 suit. But real life isn't like that. There are many issues related to changing our lifestyle that aren't as simple as keeping track of what we have for breakfast, lunch, and dinner. The discomfort we experience in changing our eating habits often has more to do with our relation to success than it does to the discomfort we feel from giving up certain foods. In one way or another, we take on a role in life. We interact with people with certain set patterns. Depending on how we feel about ourselves, we adjust ourselves accordingly. Someone who finds safety in not attracting a lot of attention may keep on weight as a blanket of protection. There may be a great deal of discomfort associated with being noticed.

Perhaps you are someone who thinks you need to always be a caregiver and put others first. Whatever is asked of you, you'll do, leaving little time or energy when it comes to caring for yourself. Others may feel that they need to fight for everything they have and find themselves in a constant state of combat. In either case, food may be the reward for a day of interaction.

The diagnosis of diabetes is a life-altering experience, and it affords us a remarkable opportunity to look inside ourselves and discover what we are all about. There's a lot more to measure beyond our blood glucose level. What should we do with this diagnosis about the way our bodies are going? We can just keep leading our lives the same way, we can panic about our lifestyle, or we can decide that this is a fork in the road and we want to reassess how we are traveling.

Some sort of reflection is an essential step in a weight loss plan. As we target lifestyle changes, we come up against all sorts of reasons why they may not be possible. So in order to achieve our goals, we must first take some time to think about these issues that might stop us. Then we can make changes from inside of ourselves—our internal life, outward to our bodies.

All of us have unexamined fears and barriers to being as fabulous as our dreams. Of course, some of us have just stopped dreaming altogether. When we set some goals for ourselves we are making a little crack in reality just by saying it is possible to make some progress. So what would stand in our way?

Ask yourself:

- What would my life be like if I were the weight I've always wanted to be?

- Do I have a secret unspoken pact with anyone to stay the same? (This could be someone from your past, such as siblings, parents, or childhood friends.)
- Could I tolerate looking great?
- Would I feel other people were jealous of my success?
- How would my loved ones react if I were thinner?
- How would weight loss change my position at work?
- Would a weight loss make me stop and consider other changes in my life?
- What else have I been putting up with in my life that I might not be happy about?
- What triggers a need to eat?

We need to find other ways to feel good besides food. Sometimes we extend ourselves for others so much that we think that we deserve a "reward." Think about how often you have had an exhausting day catering to the needs of your boss, or your spouse, or your children, or your aging parents—or, in many cases, all of the above and more. What can possibly be nicer than serving yourself a lovely piece of chocolate cake, a dish of ice cream, or a slice of pie, or some such delectable treat? Why does it feel so good? That little gift, though, will only serve to make us miserable, in health and spirit, down the pike. We need to think of new ways to treat ourselves without our previous food crutches.

Make yourself a list of those special indulgences that make you feel happy and luxurious, and post it on the refrigerator. The next time you go to indulge in food, give yourself a treat off the list instead. These treats don't have to be expensive; they just have to be special for you. Here are some I particularly enjoy:

- Sitting in my favorite corner of the house and daydreaming
- Using my special china for a cup of tea
- Enjoying a nice, hot bubble bath
- Giving my feet a good rub with body cream
- Sending an e-mail to a friend and looking forward to his reply

- Enjoying my vintage costume jewelry collection, and strategizing about where to find my next purchase
- Reading a magazine that has no redeeming merit

How to Look Like You've Lost 10 Pounds before You've Actually Done It!

Let's face it, losing weight is difficult, especially in the beginning. Yes, we are fired up with some new eating plan in hand looking clearly at the rest of our lives. Determination is written across our face, we say no to super-caloric foods with a vengeance. This is terrific, but until someone says, "Oh, have you lost some weight?" we only have our hopes for the future to keep us motivated. What do we do? How do we keep our goals ahead of us before the scale validates our resolve? The answer is to fool yourself and everyone else into looking and feeling 10 pounds thinner.

These are my tips for accomplishing this sleight of hand. Houdini couldn't have done it better. The biggest issue is *don't wait until you lose weight to treat yourself right.* Don't delay taking care of yourself.

For Women
- Buy the right lingerie that really fits.
- A proper sized bra can do wonders for your figure.
- Wear underpants that don't give you a panty line.
- Control-top panty hose will make you look like you are in control.

For Men
- Buy T-shirts that fit.
- Don't wear old T-shirts that cause your belly to stick out.
- Buy shirts that have the proper collar size.
- Buy a belt in your proper size. Throw out your old, notched belts.

For Everyone
- Buy one or two nice things that make you feel good now. How many times have you said you will go shopping as soon as you lose weight?

Men or women: don't wait! When I was at my heaviest, I ordered clothes from QVC, one of the home shopping channels. It was great. They have a 30-day return policy, I could try on things at home, and they always had larger sizes. And the price is very good. Men can find great styles at Rochester shops available all over the United States.

- Practice good grooming: well-manicured hands are good for everyone.
- Get a good haircut. It will change your face.
- Women can go to a department store and have their makeup done. Lots of times stores have special promotions where they bring in a makeup expert. Sign up to do it.
- Stand up straight. Good posture can make you look thinner—and younger.

It may seem difficult to do some of these things when you aren't feeling so hot. But you will feel so much better when you do. It's like sending a message to yourself: I'M WORTH IT. I promise it will make you look thinner and it will keep your resolve in place.

Now that you have started on a healthier eating plan, it is time to consider your exercise routine, because without exercise, losing weight is very difficult to do.

CHAPTER 5

The Body of the Future

Exercise for Vitality

A successful life plan for diabetes is dependent on several factors. The two most essential are developing a lifetime eating plan and engaging in some form of physical activity. Exercise should be a way of life, a habit that will fill you with pride and self-esteem. Raising your heart rate assists the cells in taking in the glucose from the blood. It helps work against insulin resistance.

 The Physical Benefits of Exercise

- May lower glucose levels long-term
- May lower need for medications
- Aids in weight reduction
- Helps to control appetite
- Creates more muscle mass (which in turn raises metabolism)
- Improves cardiovascular "well-being," which in turn reduces cardiovascular risk factors such as elevated cholesterol, raises HDL, lowers blood pressure, lowers triglyceride levels
- Helps raise immunity to infection
- Increases vitality
- Aids in maintaining good posture
- Aids in getting a good night's rest

Because there is such a strong link between diabetes and problems associated with being overweight, most people when diagnosed with type 2 diabetes need to reduce their weight, or at the very least, monitor their weight carefully. Exercise becomes an important component in this pursuit. You may be able to lose weight without exercise, but it's extremely difficult to keep it off for a lifetime without a physical activity plan. We need to create a "negative energy balance," meaning our output of energy must be greater than the energy (calories) that we consume during the day. Increasing our activity level is essential for this. Exercise also builds muscle mass. The stronger and bigger our muscles are the more calories we burn, even "at rest." If we build our muscles and decrease the number of calories we eat in a day, we will lose weight.

As we age, we actually lose some of our muscle mass. That means that our muscles become smaller and fat can easily become greater. Since muscles require more energy (calories) to maintain than fat, when we lose muscle the demand for calories is decreased. In addition our metabolism slows down. So when we combine these two factors with a lack of exercise we will put on weight, especially if we continue to eat as we always have. We need to counteract this trend with increased exertion.

 A Sense of Balance

As we age our sense of balance can begin to be diminished. Diabetes can contribute to this. Neuropathies or nerve damage can cause numbness in our limbs. We may no longer have the same sense of certainty of our feet firmly on the ground because of this. Diminished eyesight from retinopathy can also give us less certainty in movement.

Even if you are not experiencing a lack of balance now, it's an area to be mindful of. Yoga and t'ai chi can assist you with your balance. Light resistance exercises will also contribute to buoyancy and fluid movement.

The Mental Benefits of Exercising

Exercise has many physiological benefits, but I think just as important are the benefits to your mental health.

A physiological change occurs when you exercise. It affects your brain chemistry, which is important because heavy amounts of glucose in your blood have a negative effect on your serotonin levels, the brain chemical associated with a sense of well-being. So when we exercise we affect the same brain chemicals that are affected by Prozac and other antidepressants.

It is a rare person who doesn't have to deal with stress on a daily basis. There are types of stress that make us feel challenged and happy, but there is also the stress that raises our blood pressure and presents situations that we feel are beyond our control. In caveman days the stress (or flight or fight) we felt was useful. If a wild animal was running after us, we had the energy and automatic response mechanism to run. What do we do now when the "wild animal" is a demanding boss? Certainly we can't run or strike back. Yet our brain chemistry and physiology is left with hormones and chemicals that need releasing. That's where exercising comes into play. We are brought back to a state of homeostasis when we exert ourselves. This is the physiological state of balance of variables such as body temperature, hormone levels, and acidity levels that are ideal for the time of day, season, and age.

There's so much stress in our lives, it makes us forget about our bodies. Half the time when we are walking down the street, we don't even know how we got to our destination. Our bodies just got us there, but our minds were somewhere else. One of the great lessons of exercise is that it forces us to remember the mind-body connection.

The other day I was in an aerobics class where my peppy instructor was leading us in vigorous movements. While my body was jumping to the music my mind was obsessing about lunch. Just as I was thinking about a turkey sandwich, SPLAT! I fell right into my classmate next to me. That was a clear lesson for me to pay attention to where I was. When I

exercise and don't pay attention, the physical universe reminds me of
where I am and what I should be focusing on.

Exercise also gives us a sense of control over diabetes. It makes us feel that we are in charge. When we assign the power and decision making about our health and well-being over to others it infantilizes us. When we exercise we are taking charge of our bodies. This is something we can do for ourselves. It also sends a message to everyone around us that we care about ourselves, that we value our health.

In addition, when we exercise with others, there is a sense of camaraderie that is an essential weapon in battling the stress and isolation that can be associated with diabetes. Whether you find an exercise partner or just share a smile with the person in your aerobics class, it makes you feel connected to lots of other people. There's a wonderful sense of shared commitment to good health and well-being that connects people who work out.

Exercise: A Plan for Living

We are all told that any movement is good, that it is better to do something (anything) rather than being a couch potato. While that is certainly true, a random intention doesn't take us very far. So it's important to develop a strategy to produce results. For some of you, beginning an exercise program is a big step. For others who may already have an exercise program in place, this information here should help you keep it up. Even though you will begin to feel better after just a few sessions, remember that it takes some time to actually see measurable results. These activities will challenge your ability to stay focused and keep your goals in front of you. You won't necessarily see fast results, so you have to stick with it. Don't get discouraged and don't compare yourself to anyone else, which can be the biggest downfall in any program.

Find the Exercise That Turns You On

When you look for an exercise plan for yourself, there are several aspects that are important to consider as you build an overall program. First you need to assess what is your level of fitness. Are you new to exercise? Are you active during the day or fairly sedentary? Do you have any problems with your joints? Your feet? Shortness of breath? Start by understanding what you can and can't do, but don't use that to limit yourself—use it as a starting point. Of course, you should speak with your doctor or health professional before starting a strenuous program.

 Exercise Fantasies?

Take some time and think about activities that you would enjoy doing. Often when we fantasize and discover something we would like to do, we think of all the reasons we can't. Daydreaming can sometimes point us in the right direction. Okay, I'm never going to be in a music video on MTV, but I can take a funk aerobics class at my gym. Maybe you'll never run in a marathon, but you can train to do a walk to help promote a cure for diabetes. Don't dismiss your hidden desires.

So for those who haven't moved a muscle in quite some time, how do you get started? It can be quite intimidating and the thought of moving out of a certain comfort zone in your body may send you right to bed with a bowl of popcorn. This first step is most effectively done with a partner. Even if you start simply by walking 10 minutes a day and slowly increasing it, it's great to have another person with you. Perhaps at lunchtime you can find a co-worker to walk with you. At home, a 10-minute family walk after dinner will benefit everyone. Do you belong to a diabetes center? They often have multilevel exercise programs. It's also a good place to find an exercise partner.

Here are some activities to consider. You may find these activities at an adult education program, a Y, or at a gym, or you can do some of these in your living room.

Fifteen Choices That Will Make You Feel Great

Belly dancing

Tap dancing

Square dancing

Swing dancing

T'ai chi

Yoga

Canoeing

Martial arts

Jump rope

Jumping around to the radio or MTV

Walking with a good friend

Bike riding

Ice-skating

Swimming

Tennis or badminton

When I was diagnosed with diabetes, I decided I wanted to join a gym and really get into shape. But I couldn't do it. I was afraid that every person working out, the trainers, the people who cleaned the equipment, and anyone walking by the gym on the sidewalk would all have some judgment or opinion about me. I don't have the right workout clothes. I am too old. Everyone else is under 25 and I am double that age. Everyone will notice that I can't even turn on the treadmill let alone the newer elliptical trainer machines. I won't know where everything is.

So it took four months, from September until January, to summon the courage to go to the gym. I decided that I would try to get in shape at home first. I accelerated my exercise: walking about three miles once a week and getting on a home step machine for about 45 minutes twice a week. I also went to the video rental store and rented several different exercise tapes until I found one that I enjoyed. Then I bought it. It was great to be part of an aerobics class without having to deal with other people. I could make mistakes without judgment.

By January, I was ready. I took the plunge and went to my local gym. I swore I was the oldest, fattest person there, but by then, it didn't matter anymore because I just wanted to work out, feel better, and look good. What was the turning point? By January there had clearly been a change in the way I looked and felt. I had stuck with my new regimen long enough to have visible results. I felt mentally ready to take on the gym as the next step. I already had begun to receive positive feedback about the way I looked and I noticed that I was developing more energy and was a little less cranky in general. I also started to psych myself by thinking about the upcoming summer. I kept saying to myself: "Have the best summer of your life." This was January 1999; I thought, "Have the body of the new millennium." For me these little sayings or mantras really worked. Every time I was discouraged I'd repeat: "Have the body of the new millennium."

Early on, there were many times I didn't want to go. I would try to think of any excuse or try to find someone who would tell me it was okay not to do it. In order to push myself, I would say: "Okay, here's your choice: Either be uncomfortable now at the gym or have your toes fall off later. Which do you really think is worse?" I had to be that brutal to myself to get over my feelings of inadequacy.

Develop a Weekly Schedule

Consistency is very important. Physical activity helps maintain good control. Once you decide what you would like to do (which you can always change or augment), make a schedule of when you are going to do it. DON'T THINK YOU ARE GOING TO JUST FIT IT IN WHEN YOU CAN. IT WON'T HAPPEN. There will always be reasons not to exercise. When I first started my exercise program I'd record the workouts I did after they were completed. It was nice to look back and see my accomplishments, but it didn't help to keep me on track. That's why I recommend making a weekly schedule. It helps you stick to your goals. If a workout is already in your schedule you will know not to make another appointment at that time. Think about going over the schedule with a friend or someone at the gym if you belong to one. It helps to get another point of view and it will keep you honest if someone else is aware of your goals.

 Think to Yourself . . .

Do you look at your weekly schedule and think that you have no time to exercise? This should set off a red warning light: where is your health on your list of weekly priorities? Do you need to ask for support from loved ones or co-workers? Have you put your own needs on the back burner? Make your body and your life a priority!

When you make an exercise plan and put it in your calendar you may start to think about what time of day you are at your best for exercising. While many days we don't have a choice and must fit it in when we can, there are days where there's more flexibility. Do you feel peppier in the morning? Then try to work out then. Can you only work out at night? Just keep going. There are even exercises for people to do sitting down.

When you look at the schedule you've planned you may think you are too tired when you actually get to the gym that day. Don't give up. Exercising can actually give you more energy; you just need to get through the initial resistance. And when you are done you will feel so good about yourself that you will naturally feel peppier, or else you'll be so tired you won't care.

Make a plan and develop a consistent routine rather than worrying about being at peak physical performance. A good guideline is to do some activity or exercise a minimum of three times per week. An optimal plan for weight loss is 40 to 60 minutes, five or six times per week. Don't be frightened by this. Do what you can. In the beginning if you take a walk for 10 minutes three times a week and start building it up in 5-minute increments that is great. You should congratulate yourself for any progress you make.

Here are a few scenarios that have worked for people I have counseled:

Audrey has a demanding administrative job more than an hour from her home. Her commute required two bus rides. It seemed that exercise during the week was a challenge—or impossible. So Audrey committed herself to 30 minutes of fast-paced walking every day. Instead of taking the first bus, Audrey decided to walk the 10 minutes to the second bus stop and do the reverse on her way home. At work she set up a lunchtime walking club and clocks in at least another 20 minutes every day with a few of her co-workers.

As a young boy and teenager, Tony, a 38-year-old African American, loved football. Even as a young adult he would find pickup games on weekends at the park near his home. All the neighborhood weekend warriors would know to call him for a game. After a knee injury, Tony started to take it easy. The time he had spent playing football was replaced by television and fast food. Steadily, his muscular frame turned to pudding. The good news is that when diagnosed with diabetes, he used it as a wake-up call. He put himself on a diet and sent the word out that he was ready for a little football. As the weight came off he was able to play more and more. He also returned to his home gym and started to lift weights. Eighty pounds lighter, Tony is playing every weekend and doing weights during the week. He says there is no excuse for not working out.

Prepare Yourself for Exercise

The first thing to think about when you begin to exercise is making sure that you have proper footwear and clothing. In chapter 7, there are lots of tips on taking care of your feet. Keep this in mind and make sure you have proper athletic shoes for your activities. It's essential to make sure that you don't wear shoes that will cause irritation yet are supportive. If you are someone who hasn't worked out in a while it is best to buy shoes at a store that carries many brands so that you can see what athletic shoe fits your feet the best. Ask your podiatrist for any special recommendations, and discuss with a professional, experienced salesperson to get a proper fit in your shoe.

As for clothing, keep it simple and loose. For most of us, we just aren't interested in displaying our flesh in trendy, revealing gym clothes. I went to the GAP and bought a half-dozen black men's T-shirts. Coupled with black leotards, I feel fairly anonymous and covered.

 Special needs and thoughts with diabetes

Every time you work out you should consider the following:

- Monitor and record blood sugar before and after exercise.
- When did you eat last? Exercise 60 to 90 minutes after a meal.
- Have you had enough water? Drink plenty of water before, during, and after exercise. Remember, by the time you feel thirsty you are already a bit dehydrated.
- Have you checked your feet for sores and do you have proper fitting socks and shoes?
- Carry fast-acting carbohydrates (glucose tablets, Life Savers candy, etc.) while exercising in case of any episodes of low blood sugar.

Always Warm Up and Cool Down

Warm-ups and cool-downs are very important, and so is stretching. Don't start exercising at your optimal pace. Begin slowly for the first 5 to 10 minutes, depending on the length of your activity. Warm-up gives your muscles a chance to work better and increases your heart rate at a gradual speed. You'll be able to work out longer if you warm up slowly. Cool-down is equally important. If you stop abruptly, you risk feeling dizzy and disoriented. When I use a treadmill or other cardio machine, I decrease the pace over 5 minutes and stop. After I've turned the machine off, I take another minute to stretch right there.

Get Psyched while You Work Out

So much of exercising is mind over matter. Even people who train for marathons must overcome discomfort and resistance. As you work out, you might be overwhelmed by the feeling that you just do not want to do it anymore. At some point, everyone feels like they want to quit. But that's precisely the moment you need to keep going. As one aerobics instructor said in a class I attend, you are retraining both your mind and your muscles, so when your body says no, that's exactly the time to keep going. (Of course you don't want to harm yourself— if your body is really in pain, do stop.) But think about it: you are in a safe environment and you have set a goal for yourself, so stay focused. Don't give up. Here are a few things to think about at those times in order to stay on track. This is meant to inspire you to come up with a whole set of your own ways to remain motivated.

- I visualize my cells like a million little Pac-Man figures eating the sugar in my blood. In truth, exercise causes glucose uptake by your cells. That is one of the goals, to get the glucose from your blood and into the cells where it can be used for energy.
- Think about how you would like to look, but pick an idol that you can come close to. I am never going to be Jennifer Lopez, but I have a fighting chance at Susan Sarandon. It's great to have a visual image in mind, just make sure that you are in the same ballpark (or planet). That way you won't be beating yourself up all the time. We can really hurt ourselves with the unattainable images we see in the media.
- Sometimes when I'm on the treadmill, I imagine I'm running a marathon and my family is there at the finish line full of smiles and excitement. It helps me get over the middle of my cardio workout when I want to quit.

Consider Hiring a Trainer

This may sound like a major extravagance, but it makes all the difference to have someone in your corner. You can also get a fitness coach on a one-time basis to review your plan with you. Find one from a local gym, a Y with an athletic program, or even a local college. Ask about their certification and the training that they have had.

When you join most gyms, they give you a free session with a trainer. While this means you will spend even more money than your membership fee, it is a very good idea.

There are so many benefits to having a trainer. For one thing they can show you where everything is and how to use all the different machines. Both men and women can feel awkward trying to operate machines that they have never used before. Even if you have used machines in a gym before, they can be upgraded with new state-of-the-art technology that may not have existed when you last worked out.

Having a trainer is also like literally having a "body guard" with you at all times. You will learn how to use every machine, device, and piece of equipment in the proper way. Your trainer can design a program that is just right for your fitness level and specific body type. As you progress, they can expand your program accordingly. A good trainer can help you establish realistic goals for yourself and assist you in realizing them.

When working out it's important to know how much we can push ourselves. My trainer keeps a careful eye on me. If he thinks I am getting dizzy or faint, he has me take a break or get a snack. In addition, your trainer can become an integral part of your support system—part of the essential team. We can't get our lives under control without the support of others. I love the encouragement and sense of partnership I have had with my trainer. Time with a trainer is an excellent investment. Even if you can't afford to use one weekly, a regular fitness "check-up" is worthwhile.

Stay Active

We've discussed the necessity for a plan of action in order to produce results from your workout. As an addition to that, there are many ways to increase your general activity level. Many of these suggestions have become the mantra that we all hear: park your car several blocks from your destination; walk, don't drive; climb steps, don't take the elevator. All of this points in the same direction: a lifestyle change, an alteration in how we think about moving. There is a study that shows that people who fidget during the day in their offices stay slimmer than those who stay put at their desks. Think about how you could fidget more. *Remote control* should become a negative phrase, and it may even decrease your TV time if you know you have to get up every time you want to change the channel.

You should consider fidgeting as the first step. But nothing beats organized cardio exercise, weight training, and flexibility activities.

CALORIES BURNED WITH EXERCISE	
Activity	Calories per hour (150-pound person)
Moderate	
Walking (2.5 mph)	210
Golf	250
Swimming (0.25 mph)	300
Walking (3.75 mph)	300
Vigorous	
Ice-skating	400
Tennis	420
Skiing	600
Cycling (13 mph)	660
Running (10 mph)	900

(Adapted from *Joslin's Diabetes Mellitus,* 13th ed., 1994)

Tips on Flexibility, Weight Training, and Cardiovascular Activity

When developing an exercise program for yourself you should make sure it includes flexibility, strength, and cardiovascular workouts.

Flexibility

Flexibility exercises increase range of motion in the body's joints and keep muscles supple. Flexibility allows greater freedom of movement, improves posture, increases relaxation, releases muscle tension, and reduces risk of injury.

Some people have greater flexibility than others. It is influenced by your body type and heredity and primarily due to your gender, age, and level of physical activity. You tend to lose flexibility with age, but this is usually a result of inactivity rather than aging. Think of seniors doing yoga. Increasing and maintaining flexibility is achieved through performing stretching exercises. Stretching should be a slow and gradual process.

You should start each stretch slowly, exhaling as you gently stretch the muscle and inhaling as you relax. It is important to hold each stretch for at least 10 to 30 seconds. You should stretch to the point of mild discomfort, not pain. It is helpful to avoid bouncing while stretching to minimize muscle strains.

If a stretch hurts, do not push yourself further. Also, you should never stretch a muscle when you have not done a proper warm-up. Stretching a muscle when it is "cold" increases the likelihood of injury. The best book I've found on the subject is *Stretching: 20th Anniversary* by Bob Anderson, Shelter Publications.

Strength and Weight Training

Strength and weight training are defined as activities designed to build muscular strength and endurance, which maintains lean muscle tissue. Such exercises can be done with free weights or weight machines. Doing push-ups and pull-ups are also considered elements of weight training.

Even if you don't belong to a gym, you can do some simple exercises at home, using a book or video as a guide. A simple set of hand weights are not expensive and can be purchased in a variety of pounds. They come in 1, 2, 3, 5, 8, and 10 pounds and up. Usually hand weights are used for developing upper body strength.

Whether you use hand weights or weight machines you should set up a weight-training program or some basic routine that you do on a regular basis. A routine consists of sets and repetitions (also called "reps"). Repetitions are the number of times one lifts the weight without resting; a set is the completion of a predetermined number of repetitions (or the number of successive repetitions performed without rest).

Usually repetitions are done 10 to 12 times, and then you rest for a minute or two and do two more sets. In other words, you want to do three sets so that you end up repeating the same movement 30 to 36 times.

To avoid strength imbalances, it is important to work all major muscle groups. Your trainer can help you develop a program and learn safe techniques. More than for any other exercises, using weights or weight machines requires some instruction for optimal results. You can learn the effective methods with optimal results with an exercise professional on hand.

Some important strength-training principles include:

- Perform each exercise through a full range of motion.
- Concentrate on proper form and maintaining control.
- Avoid locking joints by always keeping a slight bend in the arms and legs.
- Use a one- or two-count on the lift and a three- or four-count on the release.
- Maintain a normal breathing pattern by exhaling on the lift and inhaling on the release.
- The last two reps should be difficult to achieve. If the last two reps are not difficult, then you should use heavier weights.

- Muscle rebuilding generally requires 48 hours, so it is best to lift every other day.
- Begin by working larger muscle groups and then move to smaller muscle groups (back, then shoulders, then biceps).

Improvement is based on the overload principle. *Overload* means that in order to improve the performance of your body's systems, that system must work harder than it is accustomed to working. *Muscle overload* means that in order to continue developing strength or endurance, the muscles must be challenged to do more.

If you are a beginner, you should start with a weight that you can comfortably lift and build slowly. Once you are comfortable with your routine, you can increase the overload by performing an additional exercise for each muscle group, increasing your repetitions, or increasing the weight by 5 percent. Some people want to build larger muscles while others just want to stay toned. This influences how much you increase your weights. In general, every six to eight weeks, you should change your strength-training program.

Aerobic Exercise Programs

The appropriate frequency, intensity, and time of an aerobic program will vary from person to person. In general, when you begin an exercise program, you should review your goals, time commitment, current activity level, and age. Next, decide how often, how hard, and how long you can exercise on a regular basis. When you are just starting out, you should focus on frequency and time rather than intensity. When you are able to exercise at least three times a week for 20 minutes, you can begin to concentrate on intensity.

Over time, the frequency, intensity, and time of the exercise program should change. To improve your physical fitness level, your body must work harder than it is accustomed to working. Physical fitness improvement can result from either a change in frequency, intensity, time, or type of exercise.

A Note about People with Special Needs

If you suffer from joint problems or problems with your nerves that affect your legs or feet, you may need to find exercises that accommodate. Consider swimming as a beneficial alternative. It will not stress your limbs, yet it will provide aerobic and strength conditioning. You can do many exercises in a chair, including leg lifts and upper-body weight training. As for equipment, try a rowing machine or stationary bicycle or a machine that has your arms move in a pedal motion.

If you are someone who is classified as obese and the suggestions listed here seem more than impossible, consider buying or renting tapes made by Richard Simmons. He is a most inspiring individual who has produced outstanding results for people who could never imagine they would ever move their bodies.

Eating for Exercise

Snacks can play an important part in any eating plan, but here are a few things to be cautious about. Make sure that you don't have a snack that will raise your blood sugar too quickly. The wrong snack could pep you up but send you crashing in the middle of your workout. If you find that you are tired in the middle of your workout consider if you've had enough food at breakfast or lunch to sustain you. Before you work out measure your blood sugar. The following chart should assist you in thinking about what your snack needs may be.

Type of exercise	If blood glucose is	Eat before you work out
Light-moderate (walking or leisurely bicycling for up to 30 minutes)	<100 mg/dl	1 fruit *or* 1 piece of bread
Light-moderate (walking or leisurely bicycling for up to 30 minutes)	100 mg/dl or above	You do not have to eat anything
Moderate (1 hour of bicycling, swimming, jogging, golfing)	<100 mg/dl	½ sandwich *with* 1 cup milk *or* 1 fruit

Type of exercise	If blood glucose is	Eat before you work out
Moderate (1 hour bicycling, swimming, jogging, golfing)	100–180 mg/dl	1 fruit *or* 1 piece of bread
Moderate (1 hour of bicycling, swimming, jogging, golfing)	180–300 mg/dl	You do not have to eat anything
Moderate (1 hour of bicycling, swimming, jogging, golfing)	>300 mg/dl	Do not exercise until blood sugar is under better control
Strenuous (more than 1 hour of bicycling, football, basketball, shoveling, hockey)	<100 mg/dl	1 sandwich *with* 1 cup milk *and* 1 fruit
Strenuous (more than 1 hour of bicycling, football, basketball, shoveling, hockey)	100–180 mg/dl	½ sandwich *with* 1 cup milk *or* 1 fruit
Strenuous (more than 1 hour of bicycling, football, basketball, shoveling, hockey)	180–300 mg/dl	1 fruit
Strenuous (more than 1 hour of bicycling, football, basketball, shoveling, hockey)	>300 mg/dl	Do not exercise until blood sugar is under better control

Low blood sugar may occur up to 24 hours after an exercise session, so it is very important to monitor blood sugar levels very closely after exerting yourself.

Snack Bars and Sports Drinks

It's hard to avoid all the advertising and promotion of sports drinks and sports bars. Every wrapper, every label, offers so many promises. Do they have any place for people with type 2 diabetes? When I read the label of many snack bars, I think I'm going to chew on a science experiment—there are so many additives. I want to eat something that has real food in it, and not chemicals. There are only two that I can recommend: Luna bars for women and Clif Bars for men. They have a nice combination of protein and carbohydrates. But don't use these as meal substitutes.

Unless you are engaging in very high-level activity like running a marathon, it's unlikely that you need most sports drinks. Have a big glass of water instead and continue to hydrate yourself while working out. If you are feeling like your blood sugar is getting very low, a small glass of orange juice or a glucose tablet will be fine.

A Word of Encouragement

Y ou need to give yourself a pat on the back for whatever you achieve with exercise. Don't diminish your accomplishments. *Any* step you take is progress. If you start on the treadmill at 15 minutes and increase to 20, that's great. Keep going. If you start by walking a quarter mile and work up to a half mile, you are making progress. If you are at the gym two days a week and add a day—so much the better. The point is that this is all progress and when you are looking at the rest of your life, every little bit makes a difference. People, when they are working out even a little bit, seem livelier. A certain kind of optimism takes over and it shows on their faces. You don't have to be at top form. That's not the point. I always tell myself that as long as I am headed in the right direction, I am doing great.

 Lost Your Footing?

Did you begin a program and then stop because of illness, injury, change in schedule, or just a fork in the road? According to trainer Michael Knowles this presents an opportunity. Don't worry about immediately exercising at the same level. Use this as a chance to take it slow and reconnect with your body. Knowles stresses that the mind-body connection is the key to a body that is toned and flexible. It's not how much we do, it's the consistency and mindful awareness we bring to the workout that makes the difference.

I was fortunate because the trainer I met at that time was a real comedian. No, seriously! He was a real stand-up comic who supported his dream during the day by being a personal trainer. Since I happen to prize brains and humor over most other human attributes, Ben and I were well matched. In our first session, we mostly talked about my goals.

I told Ben that, above everything, I wanted a waistline back (not that I ever had such a great one), but at a certain age you're lucky if you're just straight up and down and not a walking matzo ball. I also told him how quickly I was able to bulk up with muscles when working out. Ben said the activity for me was boxing. Boxing!!! I was intrigued by the idea and said I'd give it a try.

Let me tell you, I love boxing. From the first time I put on gloves I knew it was for me. It's really hard to do. And it's the most amazing workout. It develops upper-body strength and the movement is like dancing. You have to develop some internal music in order to move right.

I didn't plan to start to box, and I am not recommending it as the best exercise for people with diabetes, but I was open to it when it was presented.

Don't limit yourself. Try something new. Let yourself go. What are you saving yourself for? Try anything once. Take a buddy with you or go by yourself. Just get up and out. There is always something new to try, even in smaller cities or towns. Buy or rent a video. If nothing else turn on some music and jump around. Try a martial art. It doesn't matter what you do. You don't have to limit yourself to one kind of activity. Think of what it felt like when you were a kid and didn't have to worry so much about looking good, and just enjoyed the wonder of movement.

We didn't give ourselves diabetes. I can't imagine anyone wishing for it. There are certainly aspects of having diabetes that we can't control, but exercise is something we can control and by doing it we feel better. You can't change your genetics, but you can get up and move.

A key aspect of good control requires monitoring of our blood sugar and familiarizing ourselves with the medications available. This next chapter, combined with what we've already learned about eating healthy and exercising, is an important component of a total diabetes life plan.

CHAPTER 6

Monitoring, Medication, and Insulin

Type 2 diabetes, if caught early, can be controlled with proper diet and exercise. This requires lifestyle changes necessary to maintain a fasting blood glucose level between 80 and 120 mg/dl. This means that if your blood sugar goes below 80 or above 120 mg/dl you would take action.

The best-case scenario for a person with type 2 diabetes is to not have to take any medication at all in the beginning. This would indicate that the lifestyle choices a person has made resulted in an increase in the cells' sensitivity to insulin and the uptake of glucose in the blood.

Unfortunately, many of us can't maintain good enough control of our blood sugar, either because of our genetic makeup or because we can't make the lifestyle changes that are needed to stay in control, or our condition has progressed to the point where we need additional assistance to maintain our blood sugar. But with tight control we can make improvements. If we take medication, we can reduce it or eliminate the need for it. If we are on insulin injections, we can lessen the dosage or go back to only taking medication. There is always the possibility of better control, and the results of this, beyond the need for medication, can be quite beneficial. The more in control we are the less chance of developing complications such as eye damage, nerve damage, or heart attacks. This chapter will provide information about monitors, medication, and how to use all the related diabetes "equipment" in order to take optimal care of yourself.

In chapter 7, we will talk more about the highs and lows of blood sugar. There are physical symptoms that we can all become aware of so we feel well. But it's also easy to fool ourselves into thinking that we are fine when we are not. That is why it is so important to monitor our blood glucose levels regularly. It is the hallmark of good control.

As discussed throughout this book, tight control over blood sugar is the goal in effective diabetes management. According to Dr. Robin Goland, director of the Naomi Barrie Diabetes Center at Columbia-Presbyterian Hospital, we need to "take the emphasis off the way we control blood sugar and just make sure it gets fixed." The important thing is to avoid complications that can result from lack of control. So if you need medications and/or insulin you shouldn't place any "moral judgment" on their use.

Control is so important because the higher your blood sugar the higher your risk of complications. Think of it as a continuum from normal blood sugar (below 126) all the way up. The number actually is a marker for risk factors. Much research has shown that the chances of risk factors for complications rise dramatically above 126 mg/dl. As this number goes up, so does the chance that you will develop heart disease, kidney disease, neuropathy, eye problems, and an entire menu of other complications.

Monitoring Your Blood Glucose

The first step to gaining control over your diabetes is to monitor your blood sugar levels on a consistent basis and keep accurate records. Self-monitoring your blood glucose is a critical element in your overall diabetes care. By measuring your blood sugar on a regular basis, you know how your lifestyle is impacting your health. Recording your levels assists your doctor or diabetes educator in giving you the best care possible.

Sometimes it may be daunting to keep careful track. Depending on your personality, you may be someone who doesn't like to monitor your activities too closely. Others may find it quite satisfying to keep a careful eye on an hour-by-hour, day-by-day basis. Whatever your personal style, follow the suggestions of your health care team. Often when you are first diagnosed, you may be asked to monitor up to four times a day until you and your health care team become familiar with the patterns in your own glucose levels. For example, some people experience high glucose levels early in the morning. Others may have very high levels an hour or two after meals. Careful monitoring will help determine your glucose schedule.

And remember, the Step-by-Step Weight Loss Plan is based on monitoring your blood sugar. See chapter 4 for more details on how blood glucose levels affect what you should be eating in your diet.

> While all blood glucose meters use whole blood to measure glucose, lab equipment uses only the plasma portion of blood. Because of this difference in sample types, whole blood test results are about 12 percent lower than plasma test results.

Monitors

Your doctor or diabetes educator probably suggested a type of blood glucose meter and showed you how to use it when you were first diagnosed with diabetes. The meter may be a type your doctor works with most often, and may be computer compatible so information from your monitor can be downloaded onto the doctor's own computer. While it's important to use one that allows this kind of interaction, you may want to do some shopping around. There are many different kinds of meters out there, and all manufacturers will supply information to you if you call their toll-free number. (See the resources section.) Consult the *Diabetes Forecast Special Resource Guide 2001* for further information.

In order to assess these meters, here are some features to consider:

Size

There are meters that can easily slip into a pocket. For some, this makes a meter more user-friendly. Others who are not on the go as much may like a meter that remains firmly on a counter for easier use.

If vision is an issue you might want to look at some with larger numbers and ease in inserting a strip.

Type of Strip Required

Some have curved strips that are contoured to fit your finger. Others may feature a "cartridge" of strips so you don't need to insert one every time.

Ability to Store Information

Some can store testing date and time as many as 100 times. Additional features allow you to mark activities and mealtimes on your meter.

Computer Compatible

Some can be used with a computer program so you and your doctor can chart your blood glucose levels over time. There is a new generation of meters that will be compatible with a handheld organizer so that you can download information with greater ease. Therasense glucometers will have this capacity.

Speed

Some measure your blood in only 12 seconds. This is very good for people on the go who might need to monitor when out in public.

Precision

Most monitors available have a high degree of accuracy when used properly. It's important to test your meter once a month to be certain. Test solution is included in your starter kit. It's also useful to make special note of your reading the day you have your doctor's checkup. You can measure your monitor's accuracy against the measurement from your doctor's blood test, which will measure 10 to 15 percent higher than the one you do at home.

Alternate Site Capability

Many glucometer manufacturers now have meters that can test your glucose from a site other than your finger. After years of testing, fingertips can take quite a beating. The new meters allow testing from the forearm, thigh, and even stomach area.

Customer Care

All manufacturers have a customer support toll-free number should you need assistance.

Whichever monitor you choose, you should be aware of a variety of factors that could affect your reading. They include:

- Humidity
- Extreme light
- Touching the test strip
- Movement (taking your reading while in a car, plane, etc.)
- Dirt or lint on the monitor
- Moisture on your hands

Make sure you avoid the above to ensure accurate readings.

New Noninvasive Monitors

The FDA has recently approved the GlucoWatch, which is worn like a wristwatch. It measures very small amounts of fluid through the skin by light electrical currents. New technology is also using infrared waves.

Lancets and Lancing Devices

A lancet and lancing device come with your meter—you use this to obtain a drop of blood that you put into your monitor. Most lancing devices are shaped like pens and are adjustable to obtain shallow or deep penetration. They are relatively inexpensive and can be purchased at your pharmacy. Most have a spring action, which makes it easy to get a blood sample. Lancing devices are inserted with a lancet, a small fine object that you use to prick your finger.

When I was first diagnosed with diabetes, getting a proper blood sample was the most difficult task for me. I don't consider myself a squeamish person, but the thought of pricking my finger seemed like a dreadful task. As someone who has spent years in the kitchen, I've cut myself many times and certainly have handled sharp equipment. But my past was of no help: I simply couldn't do it correctly. I'd end up having to prick my finger several times in order to get the right sample for the meter. Tears and drops of blood would spill all over the instruction booklet. I felt vulnerable and helpless. The thought that I would be doing this for the rest of my life added to my despair.

I'll spare you the pep talk, but I will say that it does get better with repetition. This is a good reason to have sessions with a diabetes educator who you can practice with. It does make a difference when someone "walks" you through it.

When to Monitor—Keeping Records

It's very important to keep good records of your blood sugar. This will

- Allow your doctor to prescribe appropriate medications and change them when necessary
- Assist you and your nutritionist in regulating your eating plan by understanding when you have highs and lows
- Allow for greater daily self-management of your diabetes so that you can be in control
- Help you stick to the Step-by-Step Weight Loss Plan (see chapter 4)

Your team may want you to monitor up to four times a day at the beginning of your initial monitoring of diabetes in order to assess some trends in your highs and lows. Over a week's time, you'll be able to see a trend before meals and at bedtime. Common times to monitor are: before breakfast, lunch, and dinner; one or two hours after a meal; and at bedtime. If your blood sugar is in good control, you may monitor one or two times a day or as little as three or four times a week. It's always useful to monitor more when

- You are doing strenuous exercise
- On sick days
- After a particularly large meal or snack

Times to Test	Recommended Goals
Fasting (morning)	80–120 mg/dl
After meals (1 to 2 hours)	Less than 180
Pre-lunch	80–120
Pre-supper	80–120
Bedtime	100–140

Source: American Diabetes Association

Why do you need to record your blood sugar levels? It may feel like an incredible bother, but it does help to see if there are any trends. This way you will get to know your body and how it reacts to many situations, such as consuming different types of foods (especially carbohydrates, since they affect your glucose levels more than any other food) stress, and exercise. Does your blood sugar go up or down after exercise? Do your numbers change when you are stressed at work? Does a cold have an effect? Although this book is filled with guidelines, real-life diabetes management needs to be custom-made to suit your body, and you need to be in charge. With the support of your team of medical, nutritional, and exercise experts, you will learn to understand how your own body works under a variety of conditions. But it starts and ends with you. And the way you know if you are making progress is by monitoring your blood glucose levels.

Even though most monitors store your results, many doctors prefer that you keep a chart. Your health team can provide you with a booklet. One always comes with the monitor you purchase and there is usually an order form for more in the back of the log. The results you are asked to record are: date, time, pre/post breakfasttime, pre/post lunchtime, pre/post dinnertime, snack. There is also space to record insulin and/or medication. You'll find a space for notes. This is a great place to write down the exercise you did, and anything significant about your stress levels or general health that day.

Your doctor tests your blood sugar in her office every three to six months, depending on your own control and self-management. There you will have a fasting glucose test and a hemoglobin A1c test, a test that measures your blood sugar over time (three or four months). Glucose in the blood attaches to proteins (hemoglobin) present, a process called glycosylation. It remains attached until cells die off—about every three to four months. This gives an important overview of your control. The test is expressed as a percentage of glycosylation and can be correlated to your daily numbers from your own monitoring. A number of less than 7 shows that you are in excellent control.

THE CORRELATION OF NUMBERS BETWEEN A1c AND BLOOD SUGAR		
Hemoglobin A1c (%)	Average blood glucose (mg/dl)	Level of diabetes control
5.0	90	Excellent
7.0	150	
9.0	210	Marginal
10.0	240	Poor
14.0	360	

Medication

Why We Need Medication

As explained in chapter 1, when you have type 2 diabetes your pancreas makes a sufficient amount of insulin but your body cannot use it properly: your liver may be producing more glucose than needed and/or your cell receptors do not unlock to allow the glucose to enter. Depending on your blood sugar levels, your doctor may prescribe a medication to assist your body in regulating these factors. There are a variety of types of medications and they all affect different sites in the body. While people with type 2 may only take oral medication, those with type 1 are always dependent on insulin. Over time, those of us with type 2 may need to take insulin because the pancreas may slow down and could even stop producing insulin. This is when it may become necessary to have insulin injections.

There are a variety of medications your doctor may prescribe. The one feature they all have in common is that, one way or another, the goal is to lower your blood sugar. Different types of drugs work in different manners. Some enhance the effects of insulin; some work on your liver, others on the pancreas.

Here is a list of the types of drugs, their common names, and the part of your body they work on. Speak with your doctor about possible side effects of these different medications. Your prescription can be adjusted to find the optimal one for you.

Sulfonylureas

Generic Name	Brand Name
Acetohexamide	Dymelor
Chorpropamide	Diabinese
Glimepiride	Amaryl
Glipizide	Glucotrol, Glucotrol XL
Glyburide	DiaBeta, Glynase, PreTab, Micronase
Tolazamide	Tolinase
Tolbutamide	Orinase

- Work to increase the amount of insulin your pancreas makes
- Assist in having your body use the insulin it makes

Biguanides

Generic Name	Brand Name
Metformin	Glucophage

- Works on your liver to decrease the amount of sugar it makes
- Lowers the amount of insulin in your body
- Helps with weight control
- May also lower triglycerides and cholesterol levels
- Will not cause hypoglycemia

Alpha-Glucosidase Inhibitors

Generic Name	Brand Name
Acarbose	Precose
Miglitol	Glyset

- Work to block enzymes that digest starches
- Won't cause hypoglycemia when taken alone
- Taken at the beginning of a meal

Thiazolidinediones

Generic Name	Brand Name
Pioglitazone	Actos
Rosiglitazone	Avandia

- Increase your sensitivity to the insulin your pancreas makes

Meglitinides

Generic Name	Brand Name
Repaglinide	Prandin

- Fast-acting medication
- Causes the pancreas to make more insulin right after meals
- Has few side effects

We are fortunate that there are drugs to help control our blood sugar. But what is the advantage of having a small dosage or not having to take any medication at all? The primary benefit is avoiding the side effects of drugs. For example, Amaryl (which replaced rezulin) requires a bimonthly liver panel in the beginning to determine if the patient is susceptible to liver failure. Glucophage can cause some gastrointestinal problems in some, although they generally disappear over time. The fewer drugs you take or need means the less you are exposed to any side effects they may cause.

Combinations of Medications

At some point, your doctor may prescribe a combination therapy including several of the medications listed above. This is quite common because each medication contributes something different to your overall blood glucose control. It also may postpone insulin therapy. The following is a list of drugs that are often used together:

- The biguanides metformin (brand name Glucophage) and a sulfonylurea (brand names Glucotrol, Amaryl, Orinase) OR acarbose (brand name Precose) OR repaglinide (brand name Prandin)
- Sulfonylurea and acarbose

Remember that no matter what medication you take there are some standard rules you should follow.

- Read the medication labels carefully.
- Speak with your pharmacist regarding any potential drug interactions with these medications or others that have been prescribed for you.
- Check with your pharmacist regarding the storage of your medications.
- Be aware that herbal remedies can have powerful effects. Check with your pharmacist or doctor before starting a course of alternative therapy. See chapter 10 for more information.
- Ask your doctor or pharmacist about possible side effects to be aware of.
- Make sure each doctor you see knows about all the medication you are taking.

- Don't make any alterations in your medication schedule without consulting your doctor.
- If you have persistent side effects from any medication, inform your doctor.
- Do not use over-the-counter medications that contain sugar or alcohol.

Insulin

So many times when I tell people that I have diabetes, their first reaction uniformly seems to be: "Do you have to take insulin?" There isn't much editing of the fear, concern, and horror on their faces. Once I tell them I don't have to take insulin (yet), I notice a relaxation. This seems to be an emotional issue for all concerned. In many ways it is a benchmark for people with type 2 diabetes. Again to emphasize Dr. Robin Goland's message, there is no moral judgment about control. If you have to take insulin to control your diabetes, then recognize that it's a tool for keeping you healthy. It is the end result of your medical therapy that is most important—tight control of your blood sugar.

Even if you have controlled your weight, exercised regularly, and taken prescribed oral medications, you may still need to use insulin. So if you are told you need insulin, remember: anything that will help avoid complications is a blessing.

What is the formulation of insulin? What is the source of the insulin we inject? Most of the insulin we use in the United States is from recombinant DNA human insulin. It is produced from the engineering of bacteria or yeast and produces a synthetic human insulin. There are forms of insulin produced by animals, such as one type of short-acting, regular, and immediate-acting lente. This was the common form years ago but not used as much today.

Insulin with Oral Medication

For some time you may have been taking an oral medication or a combination of two. Unfortunately your pancreatic function may begin to decrease over many years by no fault of your own, and oral medication alone may not be effective enough to control your blood sugar. This is the point that insulin may be prescribed.

When you begin this course of therapy, you may need only a low dose of insulin before bed to prevent a rebound hyperglycemia in the middle of the night. This effect occurs because your liver senses that your cells need glucose and increases the amount of sugar in your bloodstream causing hyperglycemia. With a low dose of insulin, such hyperglycemia can be brought down to normal.

When your doctor prescribes insulin, you may also be given one of the following oral medications:

- Metformin
- A sulfonylurea
- Pioglitazone

Insulin with No Oral Medication

In some cases when you are first diagnosed your doctor may prescribe insulin without giving you oral medication. In this case, you will most likely take it in the morning or in the morning and evening to prevent hyperglycemia at night. Highly obese patients or those with an extreme degree of insulin resistance may need to go on insulin right away.

There are situations where your blood sugar is high but you can't take oral agents. This can occur for the following reasons:

- Acute injury, surgery, infection, extreme stress, or glucocorticoid treatment; insulin may be administered temporarily in these cases
- Pregnancy
- Liver or kidney disease that prevents use of oral medications

Types of Insulin

There are five types of insulin, categorized by how fast they work: rapid-, short-, intermediate-, and long-acting and mixtures. Other factors influence their speed, including your own body's response, the site of injection, and the type and amount of exercise you do. Careful monitoring of your blood glucose will give you and your doctor the necessary information to manage your dosage, eating, and exercise.

 Types of Insulin

■ **Quick-acting,** such as insulin lispro (Humalog), begins to work very quickly (5 to 15 minutes) and lasts 3 to 4 hours.

■ **Short-acting,** such as regular (R) insulin, starts working within 30 minutes and lasts about 5 to 8 hours.

■ **Intermediate-acting,** such as NPH (N) or lente (L) insulin, starts working in 1 to 3 hours and lasts 16 to 24 hours.

■ **Long-acting,** such as ultralente (U) insulin, doesn't start to work for 4 to 6 hours, but lasts 24 to 28 hours.

■ **NPH and regular insulin mixture,** two types of insulin mixed together in one bottle, starts working in 30 minutes and lasts 16 to 24 hours.

Injecting Insulin

There are several sites on your body to inject insulin, and your diabetes educator or doctor will tell you where the best location is for you and will explain how to do it. For fastest results, inject in the stomach. When insulin is injected in the arm, it works at medium speed, and the slowest speed is from the upper leg and buttocks. It's good to change the exact spot within the area that you inject so that you lessen the soreness that can occur from repeated injections. Regardless of the exact location chosen, insulin is injected into the subcutaneous fat, which is the area just below the skin.

It is also very important to remember that low blood sugar (hypoglycemia) can occur when taking diabetes medications, especially insulin and the sulfonylurea class of medications such as Amaryl or gly-buride. Hypoglycemia can be very dangerous and special caution should be taken to prevent and/or properly treat it. Be sure to refer to chapter 7 for more information on low blood sugar.

Storage of Insulin for Safety

According to the National Diabetes Information Clearinghouse, you should pay strict attention to the storage of insulin. For example, if you use an entire bottle in 30 days, you should write the date on the bottle and make sure it is thrown out by that date. You can keep the bottle up to 30 days at room temperature.

If you don't use a bottle in 30 days, you must store it in the refrigerator. It's important to have a back-up bottle in the refrigerator, but make sure you use it before the expiration date. Don't keep insulin in the freezer or a very hot place like the glove compartment of a car. Very cold insulin could make your injection more painful.

Before you use your insulin examine the bottle closely. Make sure it looks "normal"—no discoloration, frosting, or cloudiness should appear. If this occurs take it back to your pharmacist.

Make sure you are in regular communication with your doctor and diabetes educator about your medication and insulin. They will help adjust medicine to your needs and set up a regular routine for monitoring your blood sugar. I'd like to drive home the importance of regular monitoring. Whether you monitor several times a week or several times a day, be consistent. It will assist you in feeling in control by using it as a compass to determine many of your daily activities. Use this knowledge in combination with the tips in chapter 7 to take good care of yourself.

Taking Care of Yourself

In this book, we've spent a lot of time discussing lifestyle changes that you need to undergo in order to keep healthy with diabetes. In talking about diet, exercise, and medication, I hope that the vision of these changes are positive ones that will ultimately improve the quality of your life.

While you may be concentrating on keeping your blood sugar in control, losing weight, and exercising, it's important to think about your whole body. After all, having diabetes affects not just your blood sugar but all the systems in your body. Although you may be scared to even think about the diabetes-related complications that could happen to you, it should be reassuring and empowering for you to know that there are many things you can do for yourself, every day, to reduce your risk of complications. (Please turn to chapter 2 to learn more about the various diabetes-related complications and to find out what areas of the body can be affected by diabetes, why complications happen, what can happen as a result, and what treatments exist to help.)

The most general advice for avoiding or delaying the onset of complications is to pursue a healthier lifestyle as described throughout the book: eat carefully, exercise, closely monitor your blood glucose levels, don't smoke, and moderate your intake of alcohol. But there are more specific recommendations for avoiding complications.

Take Care of Yourself Every Day

ive stress a rest. There are really two distinct types of stress. One can make us feel more energetic and productive. We may have a lot to handle but it's all in control and we feel empowered by the experience. The other is quite different. It can wear us down and deplete our lives. Sometimes we feel pressured from the variety of situations surrounding us. It's often difficult to separate out the external pressures from work and family from the internal pressures we place upon ourselves. We may not be able to rid ourselves of it, but we can manage it. It's so important because how we manage stress affects our blood sugar. I cannot emphasize enough how important it is for us to manage stress for this reason alone. When we experience stress our bodies produce a type of hormone called cortisol, which sends extra glucose into our blood. Even though the stress may be more akin to mental anguish than fear of bodily harm, our bodies operate as if we are being attacked physically, responding by giving us extra glucose to mobilize ourselves.

Having diabetes creates its own stress, particularly when first diagnosed. While you may know that lifestyle changes will show positive results, any change that disrupts old habits can be unnerving. Learning to use a glucometer, managing new eating plans, communicating with loved ones—all can be stress producing. In addition, we can feel so vulnerable when we first get the diagnosis.

You need to look at what the triggers are for your own stress. But there are some general guidelines for management that I would like to suggest. Take a break at least once a day. Set aside any unnecessary projects. Try to find a relaxing activity to do, whether it be reading, watching TV, chatting with a friend, or going for a walk. Learn to meditate. Here are a few other ways of handling your stress:

- Write down what you are upset about; think about keeping a journal.
- Light an aromatic candle.
- Listen to soothing music.
- Do a craft project.

■ Rent one of your favorite movies, preferably an upbeat one that is going to make you laugh.

If you feel the effects of long-term stress building up to unmanageable levels, be sure to seek help, whether it be from a therapist or other professional to stop unhealthy stress from ruining your life.

Limit your alcohol consumption. One glass of wine or beer a day is fine, but beyond that, you are putting a strain on your system. If you have been used to having a lot of beer, try the light variety. If you like cocktails, try a nonalcoholic "mocktail" instead. If you enjoy meeting friends for a drink, continue to do so, just stop drinking alcohol after the first one, and then stick to club soda. For more tips on limiting your alcoholic intake, see chapter 9.

Take a walk. This is good not only for your body to get the exercise that you need but for your mental health as well. Walk your cares away. And don't let bad weather stop you. If it's too cold or hot or raining, walk around the mall, or on a treadmill or an indoor track, or put on a raincoat, grab an umbrella, and enjoy the solitude. Think about taking a 15 to 20 minute walk after every meal. It will be relaxing and help avoid dessert temptation.

Do some weight-bearing exercise to build muscle and protect your bones. Whether at the gym or exercising at home, make sure you remember to do a little weight-bearing exercise. For home use, buy some light (2- or 5-pound) dumbbells (for more information, see chapter 5), that you can use to strengthen your arms, shoulders, neck, back, and more. Also watch your local listings for exercise programs on television that may teach exercises that use dumbbells. Local video stores have exercise programs you can rent. Try a bunch until you find one that you enjoy. See chapter 5 for more information on finding an exercise program you like.

Don't sit still too long. Whether you are at an office in front of a computer or home watching TV, it's important to get up and stretch every 15 minutes. It will increase your circulation and keep your muscles from feeling stiff. Keeping constant blood flow to the limbs is something we need to be conscious of all the time.

Take a low-dose, slow-releasing aspirin once a day, if your doctor recommends it. This will help keep your blood thin, and will help prevent the clots that cause heart attacks and stroke. New research shows that it may also help to protect women from ovarian cancer. The new low-dose aspirin, sold over the counter, are much less corrosive to the stomach than regular aspirin and ensure that you don't take more than you need for the benefit. Discuss with your doctor whether aspirin therapy would be a good idea for you.

Hormone replacement therapy may be good for menopausal women. This may reduce your risk of heart disease and stroke, which increases after menopause. It can also help alleviate some of the symptoms of menopause. Talk with your doctor about whether you should be on hormone replacement therapy or natural estrogen replacements and what the risks are for you.

Avoid smoking and smokers. If there was ever a time to try to quit smoking, it's now! Try the nicotine patches or gum, now sold over the counter. Contact the American Lung Association in your area for programs that can help you quit. Smoking can contribute to heart disease as well as many other serious diseases. If you don't smoke but live around people who do, try to persuade them to renew their efforts to quit, for their health as well as yours.

Get adequate sleep. Clinical trials at the Department of Medicine, University of Chicago, have shown that failure to get eight hours of sleep per night contributes to the decrease in your body's insulin sensitivity. Chronic sleep deprivation disrupts a number of body functions.

Give your hands special treatment. Your hands are the main instruments for your body, and they do so much for you that they can easily get damaged in life's daily activities. Check your hands and around your nails for any wounds or signs of infection every day to ensure that you don't let an infection get out of control. Notify your doctor if a wound does not look like it's healing after 24 hours. Keep your hands soft and supple by using a good hand lotion, but make sure that it doesn't have any perfumes. Massage your hands (or have them massaged for you!) to improve your circulation.

Moisturize every day. Skin can get damaged easily if it is rough from being dry. A scratch on dry skin may become infected more quickly than a scratch on supple, moisturized skin. So make an investment in a good skin cream and moisturize daily after you emerge from your shower or bath. While you apply moisturizer, check for cracks in your skin or bruises, and call a doctor if a bruise or wound does not look as though it's healing after 24 hours. There are many fine products on the market, Eucerin moisturizing lotion is one of them.

Give your eyes a break. Don't strain them. If they are tired from reading or working on a small project, rest them for a while before going back to it. Make sure your diet is low in salt, as a high-salt diet will dehydrate your eyes. Wear sunglasses when outdoors to protect your eyes, which can be prematurely aged by the rays of the sun. With diabetes, your eyes are at risk for retinal damage, so any added strain on them will not be good. (For more information on diabetes-related eye problems, see chapter 2.)

Remember to brush and floss your teeth. This is an easy thing to do, but so often ignored if you are tired or busy. Believe it or not, it can help prevent heart disease and stroke, as it is believed by some scientists that bacteria that builds up from plaque and tooth decay is the same bacteria responsible for plaque buildup in the arteries of your heart. In addition, people with diabetes are at greater risk for gum infections because the bacteria thrive on the sugar-dense body fluids. Careful attention to dental hygiene will help protect against this. Make sure you see your dentist for a teeth cleaning every six months. (For more information on gum disease and other threats to your teeth, see chapter 2.)

Drink lots of fluids to protect your kidneys and other parts of your body. Fluids help rinse out impurities from your system and protect your kidneys from urinary tract infections. Drinking water also helps you to feel full, which may help cut down on too many unnecessary calories. Make eight glasses of water a goal for the day. Keep a pitcher or a bottle at your desk in order to remind yourself to drink. Make sure you are hydrated before working out by drinking a large glass or bottle of water. After you have completed exercise, replenish lost fluid.

By the time people feel thirsty they already are on the road to being dehydrated.

It's not necessary to have sports drinks or other fortified waters. This is not the source for extra nutrients. Many drinks are expensive and can be loaded with hidden sugars. Stay away from juices, as they can elevate your blood sugar. It's much better to have a whole orange than a glass of orange juice. It will provide more fiber and take more time to consume.

Carry medical identification at all times. In case of an accident, it's important to identify yourself as someone with diabetes, including what medication you are on. You can wear a bracelet, necklace, or carry a card in your wallet. Several companies make or distribute these items, including Medicool (www.medicool.com).

Take Care of Your Feet Every Day

I'm devoting a whole section of this chapter to feet. Why? Well, feet are a long way away from the rest of your body, therefore we don't spend a lot of time paying them any attention. Because of the circulation problems that can develop over time with diabetes, you may not feel little problems that develop with your feet, and if these problems are ignored, they could turn into big problems later on (see chapter 2). Now is the time to give your feet the attention they have always deserved!

Here are 10 ways to help keep your feet happy, healthy, and protected:

1. Always wear shoes and socks.

Walking around in your bare feet or just in socks, even in your own home, is a risk you do not want to take. Bare feet are at risk for treading on something sharp or banging against something, the damaging rays of sun, or any fungi from the gym. Just wearing shoes alone, without socks or stockings, could easily cause a blister. Keep your feet dry and covered when you are awake. When you are in bed, wear socks if your feet are prone to getting cold, and keep a pair of well-constructed slippers next to your bedside for when you need to get up. Make sure your slippers provide not only comfort but are thick enough to protect you from anything you may step on.

2. *Buy comfortable, well-fitting shoes.*

Spend money on your shoes to get ones that fit well and protect your feet. There are many fashionable shoes out there now that not only feel good but look good. Check your shoes for any pebbles or other objects before you put them on and make sure they don't rub up against your feet. Also, stop wearing shoes if they are beginning to thin in places. The Medicool Stretch Walker and Ambulator footware by Apex are good shoes for people with diabetes.

3. *Choose socks of proper material that fit well.*

Good socks allow your feet to breathe, protecting them from fungal infections and allowing air to circulate in case you have a wound. Some socks are seamless and are not made with elastic to further protect from rubbing and irritation. There is some debate whether to wear cotton or man-made fiber socks (*Diabetes Forecast,* January 2001). There are no scientific, controlled studies on which is actually better at moving the moisture away from your foot. However, whichever one you choose, it is wise to change your socks during the day if you perspire a lot. Make sure your socks do not bind at the top. Tight elastic will impede circulation. TheraSock, Promed, and Dura-Sox are three different brands that each offer unique features.

4. *Give your feet the "spa treatment" every day.*

Wash your feet every day, and take care to dry them well, especially between your toes. Wash your feet in warm water. There are many wonderful foot-soaking products on the market. Some are more medicinal, others are more spa-like. Either is fine. Just avoid heavily perfumed soaks. You can get yourself a foot basin for your feet. Try one with a Jacuzzi-like vibration for added decadence. Always give yourself a nice lotion treatment to keep your feet soft and smooth. Use a high-quality body lotion, such as Eucerin, mentioned above.

5. *Check your feet every day.*

At the end of the day, make sure to check your feet. You need to look for any cuts or blisters that may have arisen during the course of the day. If you have trouble looking at all areas on your feet, use a hand mirror or ask one of your housemates to help you check. Take note of any problem. If a scrape or blister does not show signs of improvement within 24 hours, call your doctor immediately.

6. *Keep the blood moving in your feet.*

Keep your feet up when sitting—this will help improve circulation. Nobody should ever sit with his legs crossed, but you should especially avoid that now. And give your toes a wiggle and rotate your feet around in a little mini-aerobic foot workout! Try this for five minutes, three times a day. Good circulation to the feet helps to avoid injury and speeds healing.

7. *Give yourself a pedicure once a week.*

Check your toenails and keep them trimmed. Trim the toenails straight across and file them so they don't have any blunt edges. It's all right to have professional pedicures, but check with your doctor if you have neuropathies. Bring your own tools to the salon to make sure that they are clean. Nail polish should be saved for special occasions only, because an infection could develop in the nail that might not be visible if it was covered by polish. Do not have a rounded shape to your nails, as this can cause an ingrown nail, which would be a big problem because of the risk of infection.

8. *Smooth corns and calluses.*

Those lumps and bumps on your feet do not help with the proper fitting of your shoes and can rub up against the softer part of your feet with the potential of scraping them. Use a pumice stone to smooth these corns and calluses after you have soaked your feet. Follow up by using your foot cream. Never use a razor or cut off calluses, which would leave you exposed to infections. Even if you have a professional pedicure, do not have your calluses cut with a razor. Consult your podiatrist for further information.

9. Protect your feet from the cold and the heat.

Be sure to adequately protect your feet against the extreme elements. Never walk on hot pavement without shoes on. Never go out without sunscreen on your feet if they are exposed to the sun. Always wear warm shoes and boots in the winter to avoid frostbite. And don't allow your feet to get cold, even if you're in bed. Wear socks to bed if your feet are cold.

10. Consult your doctor.

Have your doctor check your bare feet every time you see her. Ask for any special advice that she might have in taking care of your feet. And call your doctor immediately if any problem on your foot, such as a blister, scratch, or bruise, does not start healing within 24 hours of when you first noticed it. Take off your shoes and socks when putting on the examining robe to make sure your doctor looks at your feet every time you have a visit.

 Driving

If you are taking medication to control your blood sugar, you should check your blood sugar just before you drive, and often if you are driving long distances. Be aware of the signs of hypoglycemia (see page 136) and follow the advice below if you think you are experiencing a low.

- Pull over.
- Check your blood sugar level.
- Treat it with some juice, dried fruit, or other snack.
- Check it again before driving.

Always have a cell phone in the car if you need to call for help, and always carry snacks in your car to relieve a low. It's also important to wear a medical bracelet or have a card in your wallet stating that you have diabetes. Hypoglycemia could be misidentified as being drunk or drugged, and you want to make sure that no matter what, you get proper care.

How to Handle Sick Days

Sooner or later we will all have a sick day—feeling miserable with a cold or virus. The best defense is to have a general plan in place beforehand. These include certain guidelines to follow, such as:

1. Don't change or take any new medications until you have spoken with your doctor.
2. Test your blood glucose levels more often, at least every four hours when awake.
3. Drink a glass of sugar-free liquid every hour.
4. If you can't eat your normal foods, have a series of carbohydrate snacks every hour you are awake. They should all have about 15 grams of carbohydrates. For example:

   - 1 slice of bread
   - 6 saltine crackers
   - 1 cup of yogurt
   - 1 cup of chicken soup
   - ½ cup of apple juice

5. Consult your doctor in advance to know

   - How to determine if you should call him
   - What glucose levels are a danger sign for you (usually 240 mg/dl)
   - What over-the-counter medications you should have on hand
   - How often to test your glucose levels

6. As a rule of thumb, call your doctor when

   - You've been sick for two days or more.
   - You have diarrhea
   - You have been vomiting
   - Your glucose levels are unusually high

■ You have chest pains, dry and cracked lips, or trouble breathing

Be Aware of Highs and Lows

Hyperglycemia (high blood sugar) and hypoglycemia (low blood sugar) are serious conditions that you should do your best to avoid by learning about your own body and how it reacts. It's important to recognize the symptoms of these two conditions and how to get out of them quickly.

Hyperglycemia is a condition you are already familiar with. It's when your blood sugar is too high (above 240 mg/dl). This is the state you were in when you got diagnosed, and even when you are being treated for diabetes, it can happen if you don't keep a tight focus on your blood sugar levels and react in such a way as to lower them. The symptoms of hyperglycemia include high sugar levels on your monitor, increased urine output, and increased thirst. If you do not pay attention to your high blood sugar, it could eventually put your body in such a state that you could go into a diabetic coma (ketoacidosis), a life-threatening condition.

When you exercise, it is important to check your blood sugar about a half hour before you begin. Be aware that sometimes your blood sugar can increase because the liver, sensing heavy exertion, may produce more glucose to compensate. This is why it is so important to understand your own body and check your blood sugar frequently.

Hypoglycemia is low blood sugar, and it is characterized by feelings of weakness, tiredness, hunger, and dizziness. There are three stages of hypoglycemia and appropriate responses:

■ *Mild hypoglycemia* is characterized by shaking, sweating, hunger, and a blood sugar level around 50 to 60 mg/dl.

Treat Your Low

If you have a low, have 10 to 15 grams of carbohydrates. Consume an item off the following list:

- A sugary hard candy (8 Life Savers or jelly beans)
- 4 to 6 ounces of juice or non-diet soda
- 2 glucose tablets or 1 gel packet
- 4 packets of table sugar
- A dried fruit or 2 tablespoons of raisins

- *Moderate hypoglycemia* is characterized by fast heartbeat, mood change, headache, and blood sugar below 50 mg/dl. Double the snacks listed in the above box to treat.
- *Severe hypoglycemia* is characterized by unconsciousness, convulsions, and unresponsiveness. Emergency medical help is required. If you are with someone who has severe hypoglycemia, don't try to force a snack into her mouth, which could cause choking, but a small tube of cake icing may be squeezed into her mouth. Call 911.

You may also be irritable, sweating, have an accelerated heartbeat, feel cold, and look pale. Hypoglycemia can result from taking too much medication, delaying or skipping a meal, working out too hard, or drinking too much alcohol. The treatment is to avoid concentrated sweets at mealtime and have a series of snacks in between meals.

It is very important to recognize quickly if you are having a low, because the sooner you treat it, the easier it will be to feel better quickly. Find out from your doctor what she would consider a safe low blood sugar for you, and work to stay above it. Sometimes you can have the symptoms of hypoglycemia but it is actually an adjustment of your body to a lower but safe blood sugar level. Your body may react but when you check, it may be lower than average but not in a danger zone. If you feel any of the above symptoms or notice you are below your level when you test your blood sugar, try one of the measures above.

Make sure those around you know how to recognize if you are having a low, and how to remedy the situation. This means not only your family but your colleagues at work and those around you in your other activities. Because having a low and not treating it quickly can sometimes result in the loss of consciousness for you, it is very important that people respond quickly. Keep a snack with you at all times to treat a low.

 A Note about Hypoglycemia Unawareness

You may experience hypoglycemia and not be aware of it. Your speech can become slightly slurred, you may have a little confusion or irritability. Others will notice and you may not. This can be caused by a repeating number of hypoglycemic attacks. If you have these episodes it is particularly important that you test your blood sugar regularly during the day and when you drive.

When to Go to the Doctor and What Tests You Should Have

When you visit your doctor, blood and urine samples will be taken and sent to a laboratory. Your doctor will review these lab tests with you. But what is he looking for and why does it matter? The purpose of all these tests is to assist you and your doctor in maintaining the best control possible of your diabetes. The tests will be able to determine your blood glucose levels more exactly than your home test, as well as check your kidney function and monitor the buildup of cholesterol in your body.

With this information in hand you'll be able to answer the following questions with your physician:

- Does your eating and exercise plan support the desired level of control?

- Do any adjustments need to be made to your medication?
- Are there any complications that seem to be arising?

When reviewing the tests you will hear the following terms:

Glycosylated Hemoglobin (Hemoglobin A1c)

Hemoglobin A1c is a protein on red blood cells that can combine with glucose in the blood. When glucose attaches to the hemoglobin it is called glycosylated hemoglobin. It is measured by a laboratory test and the results are given as a percentage of hemoglobin that has been glycosylated, or combined with glucose. The more glucose in the blood the higher the percentage. The test provides a reading of your average blood sugar for two to four months. Because tests may vary with the laboratory used, your doctor will let you know what result you should be looking for.

Fasting Blood Glucose

A fasting blood glucose test measures the amount of glucose in your blood after a fast or not eating for approximately 8 to 16 hours. It is used with the hemoglobin A1c to monitor your diabetes. It's useful to take your blood sugar with your own glucometer the day you have this test done. It will give you a sense of how accurate your meter is (most meters are about 10 percent lower than lab tests).

BUN (Blood Urea Nitrogen)

A BUN test measures the amount of urea nitrogen in the blood, which is a natural product of protein breakdown and is usually excreted by your kidneys as urine.

Creatinine

A creatinine test measures the amount of creatinine in the blood, which is naturally released into the blood as your muscles move and contract. Similar to urea nitrogen, it is usually excreted by your kidneys as urine.

Both BUN and creatinine are used to monitor kidney function in people with diabetes.

Microalbumin

A microalbumin test measures the amount of albumin, or protein, in urine. Ideally, protein should not be excreted in the urine, and therefore this test can be used to monitor whether your kidneys are functioning properly. If protein is found in your urine, your kidneys may not be working as they used to.

Ketones

Ketones are a waste product from burning fat when not enough glucose is available for energy. In people with diabetes, the production of ketones occurs when too little insulin is present to allow the glucose to enter the cells. Ketones may be excreted in urine; however, if more ketones are produced than can be excreted by the kidneys, a buildup in the blood may occur. This could lead to a coma and even death. You can test your own urine for ketones as a way to monitor your diabetes.

Lipid Profile

A total cholesterol test (Total Cholesterol, LDL, HDL, VLDL, TG, Total Cholesterol:HDL Ratio) measures the amount of cholesterol and fat in the blood and encompasses low-density lipoproteins (LDL), high-density lipoproteins (HDL), very-low-density lipoproteins (VLDL), and triglycerides (TG). A ratio of total cholesterol to HDL can also be calculated.

A lipoprotein is a protein that carries cholesterol around your body, either for use by your cells or to be excreted. As cholesterol and fat are digested and absorbed, they enter your blood as triglycerides and then attach to proteins to become lipoproteins, VLDL, and LDL. These lipoproteins then deposit fat into cells and along arteries as they pass in the blood and are considered the "heart-harmful cholesterol" or "bad cholesterol." HDL, on the other hand, is a lipoprotein that picks up cholesterol from the blood to be brought back to the liver to be excreted. These lipoproteins sort of work as the reverse of LDL and are often called the "good cholesterol."

Triglycerides contain glucose and therefore require insulin to get into the cells. If insulin is limited or not recognized by cells, as in diabetes, triglyceride levels can increase within the blood. That is why your doctor gives you a separate number for triglycerides.

> The cholesterol:HDL ratio is the amount of total cholesterol as compared to the amount of HDL. If more cholesterol is present in the blood than HDL, cholesterol will be deposited into cells and arteries at a faster rate than can be picked up and excreted by HDL.

High total cholesterol levels, including LDL, VLDL, TG, and cholesterol:HDL ratio, have been found to be associated with heart disease.

Blood Pressure

A blood pressure test measures the amount of pressure placed on your arteries as your heart pumps blood throughout your body. It is recorded as the systolic pressure, or top number, over the diastolic pressure, or bottom number; for example, 120/80. The higher your blood pressure, the harder the heart has to work to get blood to every part of your body.

You should speak with your physician about all the tests listed previously, and target levels specific to you.

It's important to have these tests at set intervals. You may want to keep a log for yourself of the results.

Hemoglobin A1c	Every 3 or 4 months
Blood pressure	Each visit
LDL-cholesterol	Annually
Microalbumin	Annually
Other exams to have:	
Eye exam	Annually
Dental exam	3- to 5-month intervals

We will discuss working with your doctor further in chapter 8.

Keep Learning about Diabetes

There is new information coming out every day about why people get diabetes and new treatments that are being developed. It's always good to keep abreast of the breaking news in the fight against diabetes. An informed patient is an empowered one, and just as I hope you will benefit from reading this book, I hope you will benefit from reading more and more about diabetes and any new research that may be coming out about it.

Join the American Diabetes Association

By joining, you'll receive a subscription to *Diabetes Forecast*, a magazine filled with useful information every month. You'll also be informed about local activities, fund-raisers, and volunteer opportunities, which will give you a chance to meet other people who have diabetes while giving to the community and increasing your own awareness.

Do Research

We all learn in different ways. Some of us enjoy being detectives and seeking information for ourselves. We can spend hours searching through libraries, bookstores, or the Internet.

There are so many useful websites out there for you and your loved ones about diabetes that it would be impossible for me to list them all in this book, but many of the top ones are listed in the resources section (page 209). If you have never been on the Internet before, go down to your local library and see if they have computers available and classes in using them to get onto the Internet. As you search, remember that anyone can put up a website. Ask yourself, Is this a reliable source? Do they have an agenda that you should be aware of?

Others learn through interaction and discussion. For those who learn best this way, seminars and support groups may be useful. Some people prefer a formal professional setting, while others learn best from a peer who shares their experiences. There isn't one way to learn, but you should think about your own style and incorporate that into your own plan for mastering diabetes.

I hope these suggestions have helped you to fight diabetes. Many of the recommendations are about being good to yourself. Always remember to be good to yourself and seek the help of others, which is what we discuss in the next chapter.

CHAPTER 8

Connecting with Others

No one is in control of her diabetes without the love of those
surrounding her.   —*Carol's mother*

Coming to grips with the notion that, one way or another, we
will have to manage this chronic disease of diabetes for the
rest of our lives can be pretty startling. It's important to recognize that we cannot and should not do this alone. We need to solicit
the support of our loved ones and co-workers, as well as a team of professionals, to help facilitate our well-being. It's up to us to create this
Circle of Support.

Take a moment and visualize the people you want to include for
your support. Some may be people you live with. Then there are your
friends and co-workers. Others could be those with whom you have
very simple, yet important, interactions with on a daily or weekly basis. When I think of my circle, I visualize those around me who make
a personal contribution to my welfare.

When I start thinking that everyone in my life is disappointing me,
I know that's the moment that I need to stop and regroup and visualize these people around me in a circle, and I can see more clearly that
I am not alone. The truth is, there are always people there for us.
They may not fit the image of the way we want them to be, and they
may not even know what kind of an impact they have on our lives. But
let those people know they are important to you and your success in
living well with this disease.

I include my family members and people who demonstrate kindness to me when I think about my circle. Even the people that I have
small interactions with—like the florist on the corner who smiles
every day as I walk by, or my doorman who always has a good joke for

me—these people make a daily difference to me and I value them. Of course, these are different from the relationships we have with friends and family. But don't dismiss this kind of contact. It can still touch us. Any time we recognize another human being or have them recognize us we can have a feeling of being connected. Perhaps this is especially true in big cities where, because of the sheer number of people, it's easy to feel anonymous.

Sometimes the emotional effects of diabetes can be as debilitating as the physical ones. We need to fight the feelings of being a victim, the feelings of anger at the world for not understanding what a toll this disease takes, and overall depression. Researcher Dr. Patrick Lustman at Washington University School of Medicine in St. Louis is studying the link between poor glucose control and depression. There may even be a link between insulin resistance and depression. According to his research there may be a 20-percent greater occurrence of depression in people with diabetes than those without this diagnosis. Diabetes can make us feel separated from other people, and that isolation can have a depressive effect on our daily life. When someone shows a simple act of kindness it connects us back to more positive emotions. Interaction with others is a reminder that we are all human and have some basic desire to be connected—even for an instant. It pulls us out of ourselves and reestablishes the link to others—but we must let it happen.

So as you think about these people—those that you interact with lightly or in a more dynamic fashion—visualize what you need or want from them. Each one has an offering appropriate to your relationship. And, of course, you have contributions to make to them.

Family, Friends, and Other Loved Ones

Before we can ask much from others, it's a good idea to take a deep breath and try to organize ourselves in adjusting to this lifestyle change. First, we need to see how we've been affected by the changes required in our lifestyle. Make an assessment of the physical changes you may need to take and the emotional changes you're going through. For instance, are you intimidated by the idea that you should exercise now to keep your diabetes under control? Or do you hate the idea of eating a diet different from those around you?

Second, notice how these important changes impact members of your family. Are some more affected than others? Do some have concerns they need to express? They too will have to make adjustments at home. In the case of dietary changes, it may not be desirable for you to encourage everyone in your house to eat in a new way. Would your family be willing to eat a new healthy diet the way you want to do?

Here are some suggestions on how to get your family and friends into your circle of support:

- Give them materials about your diagnosis (books, pamphlets, websites—see the resources list, page 203).
- Take them with you to doctor's visits.
- Have a regular family-and-friends meeting (this is especially helpful in the beginning), where you explain what is going on and what needs to be done.
- Send e-mails about what is happening and what can be done.
- Take them with you to lectures and information sessions.

Over many years, I've observed the effect that my mother's diabetes has on our entire family. With four siblings and a chorus of young people from the next generation, our family gatherings can have a circus-like atmosphere. But no matter how joyful the jamboree, if my mother is not well, we all feel the effects. She used to love to tap dance and would perform a little jig to the delight of everyone. Now, when her blood sugar is out of control, even coming to the dinner table is an effort for her. None of us wants to celebrate at those times. We want to do whatever we can to make things better for her, but we often feel quite helpless. I wish my mother would tell us what to do.

So how can we reach out to our family and friends in order to have them rally around us? A first important step is to simply ask people for help. You may find it so hard to communicate your needs and fears, but if there is ever a time to do it, it is now! Let everybody know that you need help in changing your lifestyle, and it's likely that they will make a good effort on your behalf. Most people love to be wanted, and to be useful, and to help make a difference, and they only need to be asked to get them going. Many people don't want to "interfere" in your life, and so are hanging back until you ask them to get involved.

At first you may not know what it is you need help with. These changes are all so new. Listed below are activities that many people find helpful to ask from their loved ones. You can use this as a springboard to think about and communicate what it is that you really want from those around you. The more you can formulate concrete requests, the more you give others the opportunity to rally to your aid.

Some Supportive Activities for Friends and Family

- Have everyone adopt a healthy eating plan at home
- Clear the house of temptations (or at least don't flaunt them) like candy and snacks
- Join with you in athletic activities
- Make sure you have the time to exercise
- Help to keep you on an eating schedule
- Learn the signs of low blood sugar and what to do about it
- Help set up a system for taking your medication
- Give you a chance to complain once in a while
- Keep a calendar of doctor visits, trips to the gym, the nutritionist, etc.

Some of us can handle intrusion into our lives more than others. There may be areas where you want some "tough love," and other areas of your diabetes management where you need to have a little room. We have to take the lead and give cues to our loved ones. Be aware that, as in all aspects of family life, support can have its ups and downs. Keep your friends and family informed of your needs as they alter or develop.

I've asked a number of my friends and family if they would like to have their blood sugar checked. I go through the entire process with them of drawing a drop of blood and using the glucometer. This may sound gory, but it gives them a sense of what I have to do every day. They also can see what their levels are and see whether their numbers are looking high and are at risk for diabetes.

If You Live Alone

When we live with other people, we need to adjust ourselves to their needs as well as our own. When we live by ourselves, we can make our own schedule, which is often more orderly. We don't need to include the agendas of other people in our daily plan. So barring unforeseen circumstances we can decide when we want to eat, sleep, and exercise without considering the needs of other people. However, living alone presents challenges and it's important to be aware of them.

Here are some points to consider when living alone:

Bingeing on food or not eating enough of the right things: Nobody will catch you if you are eating badly or not following your recommended eating plan. While this might make you feel better in the short term, it will not help with your long-term health. If you are having trouble with either or both of these problems, make sure you talk to someone about it. Try to examine what is causing your problem. Perhaps merely thinking about eating by yourself takes away your appetite. On the other hand, for those of us who overeat, the very idea of being alone is so anxiety producing that food becomes our friend and comfort. We can get so obsessed with food that it takes up that lonely time. Eating poorly is a downhill spiral. If you find you are developing bad habits, do your best to change them. If keeping a food diary is too difficult for you, try to keep a checklist of the categories of food you've eaten on any given day. (See chapter 4.)

Being unaware of low blood sugar: It is easy to be oblivious to lows when you are by yourself. With no one around to recognize your low blood sugar you could have hypoglycemia and not be aware of it. (See chapter 7 for more about hypoglycemia.) It's useful to have a chart of the warning signs posted inside your medicine cabinet or kitchen cupboard just to keep you aware.

You may be unaware of bruises or infections: It's hard to see every place on your body, and living alone, you do not have the advantage of having someone who can check them for you. Make sure you have a full-length mirror in a brightly lit room, and a handheld mirror to check your feet and other areas (see chapter 7).

Having to generate physical activities on our own: If you are prone to goofing off or avoiding exercise, it is imperative for you to stop this habit! Sure, you may have a friend who goes with you to the pool on Mondays for a swim, but nobody else may know that you aren't doing any other exercise for the rest of the week. Be sure to enlist a person who knows you very well, and knows when you are lying, to check in with and report that you've been doing your exercises. Another problem is that you may be disciplined about working out but may find it lonely to do it on your own. Try to make working out a social activity if you find yourself feeling that way—join regularly scheduled classes or have exercise buddies whom you can count on to always be there for you. Here's a tip: In your date book or wall calendar, make a check mark every time you work out. It helps to keep you from fooling yourself.

Lacking in a safety net: It's doubly important to reach out to others so there will be somebody who knows how you are doing on a day-to-day basis. Let a friend, neighbor, or a nearby relative know about your condition so they can check in on you if they don't hear from you or see you. Let them know if you're traveling, so they won't worry if they can't reach you. Or, set up a buddy system with another person who has type 2.

Joining a Support Group

As we have seen, there are many avenues for looking after your-self. But sometimes it's useful to be with other people who are up against the same or similar challenges that you face. Support groups can be very effective. I ran groups at New York University for the faculty and staff with type 2 diabetes. Some of the benefits people report from this experience are:

"I feel like I'm not alone."
"It's nice to see how other people solve problems."
"I learn how to deal with family and friends."
"A group helps me stay motivated."
"It's a way of reducing some of the stress I feel."

There are many kinds of support groups available. Some are for specific needs and populations, while others are more general. You can find them through your health care provider, diabetes center, or local chapter of the American Diabetes Association. Diabetes educators, nurses, nutritionists, social workers, and mental health professionals can run groups. If you are homebound or want additional support, you can find online chat rooms dealing with specific issues (see Resources).

So what can you expect from a group? First, groups should always have an atmosphere of safety and free expression. In groups I ran at NYU, I had some ground rules: we don't criticize anyone for the way they feel, we don't interrupt, and we don't repeat information we have heard in the group to anyone outside the group.

Individual problems, especially on a large scale, won't be resolved, although a group can be a wonderful catalyst for action. With this in mind, I heartily recommend groups. It's a great aid, especially in the beginning of your management, and can serve as a safety net throughout and reenergize those veterans who may experience some burnout.

Getting Your Professional Team Together for Mind, Body, and Spirit

As you work with your family, friends, and coworkers, you also need to reach out beyond them to create a team of professionals for your healthy lifestyle. Imagine that you are an Olympic athlete vying to win the gold medal in the marathon. You need to get your coach, your nutritionist, your sports psychologist, your fund-raisers, your travel agent, etc., all lined up to help you with your quest for the gold medal. Consider your living with diabetes as a kind of Olympic marathon race, and get that team assembled.

Who Should Be on Your Team

Most likely you were diagnosed with diabetes by your primary care physician. It is with this doctor where you will set the cornerstone for controlling your diabetes. However, there are other people to assemble in order to make sure you manage your diabetes head to toe, inside and out.

In thinking about your team of professional supporters, this is a good time to envision how *you* want to be supported. Are you someone who enjoys a great deal of personal interaction or do you want people whose professional knowledge is available only when you need it? In some cases, you'll need some intensive contact in the beginning to set you on the correct path, then you may just want to be able to phone or visit them if you have any problems or questions. For example, you may need to work with a nutritionist to set up an eating plan. If you need to lose weight, you may want to continue weekly sessions until you've mastered the plan and subsequent pitfalls. After that, monthly sessions might be useful.

Doctor

You should have one physician who is the point person for all information and tests. This could be your family physician, internist, endocrinologist, or whomever you consider your primary care physician. The main issue is having a good relationship with your physician. Although most doctors have less and less time for individual patients these days, there are some doctors who make sure patients can reach them, even with questions that might appear to be "dumb." My doctor hands out a brochure to every patient urging them to call with questions. He also has a website filled with up-to-the-minute information and a system to post questions off-hours.

 Tips for Visits to Your Doctor

- *Be prepared.* Make a list of any questions you might have. Take some time and go through your body from head to toe. You might even want to go over the list with a family member before the visit. Make sure you know what tests are going to be done so that you know whether to fast or not.
- *Bring your meter and record book.* Your doctor will want to know about any highs, lows, or significant trends in blood sugar levels.
- *Take off your socks.* This is a gentle reminder for your doctor to check your feet.
- *Have special concerns? Bring a family member or friend with you.* With so little time for each patient, physicians often have to give information quickly. Bringing someone with you will help later in remembering what was said.
- *Take notes.* It's useful to keep your own record of each visit. Think about recording your visit.

Almost as important as the doctor is his support team. If your doctor has a warm and efficient front office staff, they can make sure you get your questions answered, and they often act as a guide for referring other services.

While you may be able to get basic quick questions answered, most doctors are not set up to give you the full spectrum of diabetes education you need. We cannot rely on them for all our diabetes education or management. It's useful to get some recommendations from your doctor to enlarge your health care team. Most likely the hospital with which your doctor is affiliated will have a diabetes education center. From there, you can locate a number of team members that you will need.

Is Your Doctor Right for You?

1. Does the doctor suit your style? For example, do you prefer a quiet doctor, a doctor with a sense of humor, a dynamic doctor? Note: If you feel that your doctor is judgmental of you, find someone else. You have a right to feel empowered by your experience, not diminished.

2. Does the doctor operate in a group practice? How often will you get to see your own doctor?

3. If you have an interest in alternative therapies, is your doctor willing to consider them and support your decisions?

4. Does the doctor have a good office staff? Are they courteous and pleasant to you and get you the doctor in a timely fashion when you need to speak to her?

5. Does the doctor's office deal well with your insurance company's paperwork? If not, you may have to do more work than you bargained for in getting reimbursed.

6. Is the doctor affiliated with a hospital that you like? This is most likely where you'll be admitted if you have a problem that requires hospitalization.

Endocrinologist

When and why would you seek the help of an endocrinologist? There may come a point where you feel you need more specific attention, or your primary care physician may even recommend it. An endocrinologist has specialized in the complex hormonal systems of the body. Many endocrinologists have a subspecialty of diabetes. Ask the doctor what percentage of the practice is devoted to diabetes.

See an endocrinologist when

- You have not been able to get your blood sugar levels under control while seeing your primary care physician
- You develop complications of diabetes (as outlined in chapter 2)
- You have questions and concerns not dealt with by your primary care physician

Pharmacist

More often than not, the little corner pharmacy you once used to visit has been supplanted by a large chain drugstore that sells everything from diet soda to cleaning products. Somewhere in the back of these stores is the pharmacy. The bad news is it all seems less personal; the good news is these large stores have the ability to provide a great deal of information to the customer. They can often give you useful printed material on a prescription that comes from their database and includes information about precautions, side effects, and other warnings. Large pharmacies often have a very large selection of diabetes products.

But big or small, pick one pharmacy and stick with it. You want to have all your medications listed in one place so that someone can monitor your drug interactions. Even at a chain pharmacy, introduce yourself to the pharmacist, who can advise you on your medications and on the effects of over-the-counter remedies. A pharmacist is a highly trained professional who should be able to answer all of your questions about how and when to take your medication, and should be available to take your calls and follow up with your doctor if there is any discrepancy.

Nutritionist

When you are first diagnosed, you may be referred to a nutritionist, since good nutrition is such a vital component in staying well. This is a person schooled in the effects of food and nutrients in your body, and who will be able to help you create a successful eating plan in order to raise your energy and lose weight if needed. Ask your doctor or diabetes care center for a referral or you can call the local chapter of the American Dietetic Association.

Diabetes Educator

Diabetes educators are a group of people—nurses, doctors, nutritionists, and others—who specialize in the treatment of people with diabetes. They help you learn to live a healthy and productive life with diabetes. Many of them work in hospitals with patients, or they may work with individuals. They also may be found in doctors' offices, nursing homes, and neighborhood clinics. A diabetes educator can be there for you when your diabetes is first diagnosed to help you learn the new skills you will need. Look for the initials C.D.E. after the name to indicate a person who has met the certification standards.

Anne E. Daly, M.S., R.D., C.D.E., President-Elect of Health Care & Education, Board of Directors, American Diabetes Association, offered some pointers on finding the C.D.E. that's right for you.
- Interview the C.D.E. and make sure that your personalities fit.
- You should feel the C.D.E. creates a rapport so you are comfortable asking questions.
- You can ask how many patients the C.D.E. has and how often she is available.
- Be up-front with the C.D.E. about making lifestyle changes. Don't make promises you aren't going to keep.

Contact the American Association of Diabetes Educators to find one near you (see the resources list on page 203).

Podiatrist

It is very important to get a good recommendation for a podiatrist. A foot doctor will take care of any structural problems with your feet that might lead to infections or other problems down the road. A podiatrist is a specialist in dealing with the foot, and should be seen yearly or if you experience any problems.

Dentist

Make sure your dentist is aware of your diabetes. It's advisable to have your teeth checked frequently, at least every four to six months. If you notice any mouth sores, let your dentist know right away and get them treated quickly.

Eye Doctor

Your eye doctor should be made aware of your diabetes and be well versed in the issues of diabetic retinopathy. Your ophthalmologist or optometrist should regularly examine you for the early warning signs.

Exercise Physiologist

If you join a health club, you very often can have a free session with a personal trainer. Personal trainers should be certified by ACE (American Council on Exercise). Some trainers are also exercise physiologists. In order to set up a complete and balanced exercise program for yourself, you may want to meet with one. This is a person who has a master's or doctoral degree in exercise physiology and should be certified by the American College of Sports Medicine. This is especially important if you have specific knee or joint injuries or limitations, or have suffered from a heart attack or stroke.

Spiritual Adviser

As you may have already discovered, diabetes has a major impact on every aspect of life. The care is not isolated to a prick of the finger or an oral medication. If there is one message in this book it is that diabetes care affects the total person—the mind, body, and spirit. Each aspect is essential for us as human beings and we need to be mindful of each aspect for total care. You may have always enjoyed a rich spiritual life with your church, synagogue, or other place of worship. This can be a wonderful support system, whether simply experiencing your connection to a community of like-minded folks or by drawing on the inspiration of a religious leader. As with many other aspects of this diagnosis, you can use this as a time to reevaluate your priorities and discover whether you can draw on a spiritual life. If you are searching for a group with which to align yourself, there are many avenues to try. Of course, word of mouth is useful. Also, many spiritual and religious groups have open-house evenings. There are centers in many cities, such as the New York Open Center, that present a variety of points of view, one of which you may find gels with your belief system.

Mental Health Professional

Diabetes can be stressful and isolating. Unfortunately we can all face some degree of depression at some point. It's important to have someone to speak with who is outside of our friends and family, someone who can listen without judgment and is not personally invested in what we have to say. There are people available with a variety of credentials: MSW, psychologist, and psychiatrist. You can ask your physician for a referral. Many universities and teaching hospitals have training programs for graduate and doctoral students in mental health that offer supervised therapy on a sliding scale.

After reviewing all the ways you can connect with others for your support, I would like to suggest moving the energy in the opposite direction. Try doing some volunteer work, especially for the American Diabetes Association. Sometimes it is such a relief to get the attention off of yourself, even (or especially) when it feels that you aren't getting enough consideration of your own. When you do something for others, you may not immediately have a rush of good feeling. It could take time, but it will be worthwhile. However, if we are discussing connecting with others, it really doesn't matter in the end who makes the first step or who is doing a "good deed." What counts is the very act of connecting. And when you do something for others it creates a bond. And one could even question who is really the giver or the receiver.

Connecting with others requires being able to participate in outside events and family occasions. To learn more about the ways we can do this in a healthy manner, continue on to chapter 9.

CHAPTER 9

Real-Life Suggestions for Eating Out and Special Events

Having diabetes doesn't mean you have to give up those things that you most enjoy, such as eating out in restaurants, visiting friends and family, and traveling. You want a full, active life for yourself, and it's important to incorporate those needs into the way you live with diabetes. Since we have to manage our diabetes for life, it's important to master certain modes of behavior so we don't feel constrained by this disease.

Living the good life while responsibly living with diabetes requires some navigation, but it's so important to make this mixture work. The more you can create positive modifications to your lifestyle, the more you will feel in control. And with diabetes, being in control is both a physical and mental state. Mentally, it's good to know that you can be presented with new situations and that you'll know you have done the utmost to keep yourself feeling physically healthy.

In a sense, we are choosing a healthy lifestyle and our diagnosis was the wake-up call. We don't want our lives to be run by diabetes. The goal is to have a life that incorporates our needs. Otherwise the disease can turn into a monster we are carrying with us wherever we go.

I have found that when it comes to going outside your own controlled and ordered world, a successful foray will take dedication to your well-being, a gentle but firm attitude with others, and a bit of planning. Let's see where the pitfalls are out there and how you can enjoy yourself in all situations while sticking to your plan. With a little forethought, and armed with the tips in this chapter, you can enjoy life's pleasures and still maintain your healthy new lifestyle.

Eating in Restaurants

If we could all eat in a highly controlled environment at home and never venture forth, we might do quite well following our chosen food plan. However, that's not real life. We're all faced with both delightful and tension-filled situations where food plays an important role. It's very satisfying to be able to enjoy yourself and at the same time make sure your health and well-being aren't compromised. Let's look at some issues and strategies.

When I was first diagnosed, I had a lot of anxiety about eating out in restaurants, especially as it makes up such a huge part of my life. You see, living in New York, I dine out many times during the week. It's hard when you are trying to establish new habits to break your routine, and restaurants are the ideal place to fall prey to temptation!

Here's what I discovered: Most restaurants are not built for people on special diets. Mass-market establishments are designed to feed as many people as possible. There's little room for individualized needs. Other restaurants are theme-driven and the theme is rarely a "special" diet. Very high-end restaurants are often serving food that highlights the chef's techniques and self-expression.

What's the most practical way to deal with eating in restaurants? How do you choose a restaurant that fits your needs? Much depends on two factors: the type of restaurant you are visiting and the degree of hospitality a restaurant creates. You can't determine this by price or ethnicity of an establishment, but by how flexible or accommodating the staff will be. A higher-end establishment, one would hope, would be more obliging in return for the price you are paying. But that's not always the case.

According to food authority Mimi Sheraton, restaurants should be able and willing to make certain substitutions on any meal if you ask to switch something that is easily available in the kitchen and of comparable price. For example, if you see plain spinach listed several times on a menu and want to substitute that for the heavily buttered mashed potatoes, the restaurant should accommodate your request.

Of course, if a dish is made in advance and can't be altered, there's little a restaurant can do except offer other suggestions.

If I find a restaurant is not willing to oblige, then I won't continue to go there. Again, it is a question of hospitality, not price. If a restaurant has an adversarial attitude toward customers, then they don't deserve your patronage.

Help from the Staff

Many times I have found that a good experience dining out has more to do with the interaction with the wait staff than anything else. Whether in a diner or four-star establishment, they have the capacity to set the tone for the entire meal. They should be hospitable whether a customer is on a weight loss plan, has food allergies, or, as with diabetes, has some very definite restrictions. It's their obligation to know what the ingredients are in the dish or be willing to find out for the diner.

Frequently, if I alert the waiter that I have a medical condition that doesn't allow certain food, I get very good service. If you would rather not reveal this information or other intimate details to this gentleman or lady, you should be able to just ask some basic questions in order to determine if a dish is right for you.

Here are a few pointers when dealing with the wait staff:

1. Be friendly, and remember you're asking for something out of the ordinary from them. Don't act like you are entitled to special treatment. Remember, just as you want an aura of hospitality and cooperation, so does the restaurant. You'll get a lot more out of them with your own good attitude.
2. Don't rely on the waiter to know what is good for you. Have some questions in mind.
3. Tell the waiter what your parameters are and ask if there's something he can suggest.
4. If you see something that looks good on the menu, you can ask the waiter if it fits in with your needs.

5. It's okay to ask a waiter to question the cook or chef about the ingredients.

What to Order?

Main Course

It's important to start with your main course, and then fit the rest of the meal around that choice. I look for something that is simple: let's say, roasted chicken. If I ordered beef, I would want to be certain that it was a lean cut (sirloin or filet mignon as opposed to porterhouse). I avoid any dish that's made with fruit and certainly anything glazed with sugar, honey, etc. The dish might have a nice sauce to accompany it. If I suspect the sauce may have a lot of butter or cream, I don't order it unless I can get the sauce on the side. Very often, I can have a small amount of a sauce as an accompaniment without having to have the whole amount that would normally be served with the food.

In general, look for food that can be separated into parts—meat, sauce, and vegetables. There are many restaurants that now present food in a vertical fashion. For example, a chicken breast on top of potatoes with spinach in between, covered with a sauce and garnished on top with some crispy fried julienned vegetables. Every food group should be in its own corner—ask for it that way. Then you will have more choices about what to eat and how much.

When ordering, you may want to think about ordering a salad and another appetizer for your entrée. They are often varied and big enough to give you a complete meal.

If you are in a situation where there is nothing that fits your plan, then just think in terms of portion control (something we should all be concerned about, no matter what). Have a smaller portion of whatever is presented.

Healthy Choices for an Entrée
- Roasted or grilled chicken
- Grilled or poached fish
- A shrimp cocktail and grilled vegetables
- Grilled vegetable platter
- Lean meats—look for sirloin cuts
- Soup, salad, and a side dish
- Several healthy appetizers

Ask about the portion size before you order. A 3-ounce portion of meat is about the size of a deck of playing cards. A serving of baked potato is about the size of a computer mouse. Do the vegetables have oil or butter on them? Keep visualizations of measured portions in mind.

When eating out, avoid food that is labeled "fried," "battered," "breaded," "au gratin," "creamed," "scalloped," or "Alfredo." Look for menu items that are roasted, poached, grilled, or broiled.

Think about splitting an entrée with a friend, or split it for yourself and take half home as a leftover. Ask about the preparation of the food and know that you should have it if it's been broiled, baked, poached, or grilled. Avoid fried food.

Love cheese? Instead of having a dish filled with cheese, order a salad and have a little Parmesan grated over your dish. It will give you the taste without all of the fat.

If you order baked fish, ask if it's stuffed. If it is a bread stuffing, it will most likely also have a good portion of fat in it. Either eliminate the stuffing or adjust for it by forgoing bread or another starch during the day.

Order a vegetable side dish without oil or butter on it. If that's not possible, try to pull the vegetables out of the butter or oil.

Appetizers

Next you need to think about the appetizers. Should you get one? Appetizers can be very dangerous, because in many restaurants they are more interesting—and more full of fat—than the main dishes. It's a course where chefs sometimes go wild with creativity and calories. Stick to a soup (without cream or butter in it) or a salad. This cuts your hunger without doing harm. When I order a salad, I have them put the dressing on the side, or ask for oil and vinegar. You haven't done much good for yourself if you have a salad with lots of dressing on it! Remember, when fat is taken out of a food, so is much of the flavor, so a "low-fat" dressing can have a treacherous amount of sugar added to it for flavoring. Avoid a salad drenched in a dressing.

Beware of the Bread!

The big issue from the moment you sit down at your table is the bread—hot, steaming, and freshly baked. It's very tempting. But even the most nutritious bread can add hundreds of calories to your meal before you even get to the appetizer. Make sure that you think about how much starch you've already had that day and if it fits into your basic plan before giving yourself a green light for some. If you can't handle the temptation, have the waiter remove the entire basket of bread immediately. Another choice is to have some bread but scoop out the center where most of the softness and calories are, and eat only the outside crust. Save those calories for something later. And it's best to lose your taste for butter on bread. Even a little pat of butter has 45 calories, and it's all fat.

Dessert

When I was first diagnosed, I found dessert time particularly difficult, since in the beginning I didn't even want to tempt myself with a spoonful of sweets. I was afraid that one bite would lead to another and off I would go, forgetting my resolve. "Just say no" has taken on new meaning for me, and it applies to desserts! Much of this has to do with breaking old habits. It's pleasant to have something after dinner, but when first diagnosed, it felt better when I didn't have anything. I also could use that time to think about why I wanted the dessert in the first place. Was it a reward for something during the day? Did I want to be like everyone else at the table? Was I pretending I didn't have diabetes?

Often, I felt awkward when the waiter included me as he passed dessert menus around to my fellow diners. I wondered whether to read it with interest, and thus imagine those rivers of chocolate or mounds of confection waiting in the wings. What do I say when my dining buddies discuss which desserts look good? They would query: Should we share or get "something for the table"?

I was never a big dessert eater, but after I was diagnosed, I missed the camaraderie that desserts create when you dine out. I've since gotten over it. Depending on my mood, I say no thank you when a waiter asks about dessert, or if handed a menu, I just leave it where it was placed.

If you do want to enjoy the experience of lingering after a meal, order a cup of tea or coffee. And if that alone doesn't satisfy you, and you really want dessert, you should be able to have some on occasion. Just make sure it fits in your plan for the day. Here are a few suggestions:

1. Skip the bread before dinner.
2. Eliminate the potatoes or other starch in your main course.
3. Skip one fruit serving during the day.

4. Cut the portion in half or share it.
5. Limit the number of times a week you do this.

Menus

It's important to be able to eat many different kinds of food, because whatever your eating plan, it should be one that you can be on for life. Being able to enjoy food is one of the great pleasures, especially when coupled with socializing.

The overall trick is to get the best flavors of each cuisine without all the calories or fat. Generally, adding lots of vegetables is most helpful. And, of course, try to keep the sauce on the side.

I have chosen a few ethnic cuisines that are popular with most diners and can provide some very unhealthy hazards for the diner with diabetes. Listed below are what you can safely order and what should be avoided.

Chinese
Order
   Steamed vegetables
   Brown rice
   Poached or steamed fish
   Roasted Cantonese chicken
   Soups with clear broth
   Request stir-fry with little oil or mix stir-fry with steamed veggies

Avoid
   Fried rice
   Fried noodles
   Fried dumplings
   Anything labeled "crispy"

Note: Most Chinese dishes are cooked with sauces filled with hidden sugar. When ordering, ask the waiter to cut down on the sugar and fat. Since all dishes are made to order, they should be able to fulfill your request.

Italian
Order
> Cioppino or zuppa de clams (fish soup)
> Grilled fish
> Marinara sauce

Look for Terms Such As
> *alla griglia* (broiled)
> *bolliti* (boiled)
> *sènza sale* (without salt)

Avoid
> Breaded veal dishes
> Dishes layered with cheese (use Parmesan sprinkled on top for a cheese flavor)
> Creamy sauces like Alfredo sauce

Mexican
Order
> Fajitas (pan-seared vegetables and chicken or beef)
> Black beans and rice
> Soft tortillas
> Baked enchiladas
> Salsa

Look for Terms Such As
> *A la parrilla* (broiled)
> *Al vapor* (steamed)
> *sin mantequilla* (without butter)
> *Sin sal* (without salt)

Avoid

Quesadillas

Guacamole with sour cream (a half cup of guacamole alone is at least 200 calories)

Refried beans

 Healthy Food Claims

What does it mean when you see the claim that food is "healthy" on a menu? In 1996, the Federal Drug Administration created a regulation that requires "restaurants to support nutritional claims made on their menus." Terms such as *light, low fat,* and *sugar free* can only be used if there is a "reasonable basis" for the claim. Restaurants need to justify all statements with either a recipe or nutritional analysis.

Alcohol

A Few Guidelines

Discuss with your dietitian or diabetes expert the way you can incorporate a drink into your eating plan. You metabolize alcohol like fat, so one alcoholic beverage is considered two fat servings on the exchange system. The American Diabetes Association recommendations are for no more than one drink per day for women and two drinks per day for men. (One alcoholic beverage is 12 ounces of light beer, 5 ounces of wine, or 1½ ounces of distilled spirits such as vodka, whiskey, gin, etc.)

Let your doctor know if you drink, so that your medication can be adjusted.

Here are some tips on drinking alcohol:

- Check your blood glucose before you drink. Make sure you are under control or don't even have one glass.
- Savor your drink. Slow down and have just one.

- If thirst is your main concern have water, sparkling or plain, first. Don't use your drink to attempt to quench your thirst.
- Mix wine with seltzer for a wine spritzer. This will stretch out your drink and cut the alcohol.
- For other mixed drinks, use diet drinks including diet tonic water if available. Mixers can add lots of sugar.
- It's best to have something to eat with your drink. Try vegetables or low-fat snacks like pretzels. Avoid high-fat hors d'oeuvres and nuts. Drinking can loosen your resolve to eat healthy.
- Don't drive after drinking.
- Make sure you carry some identification that you have diabetes.

Lunchtime and Snack Time Strategies

I'm always concerned that I'm going to be too busy to stop for lunch or a snack. When that happens, I can feel my blood sugar go down (so can everyone around me). I get very cranky. I'm sure we all have battle stories related to this. In order to avoid the concern I keep a little drawer full of emergency rations at my desk. Some of these items also find their way into my purse if I am out and about all day. See if these work for you:

All-natural "cup of soup"
Vanilla soymilk (available in aseptic containers, no refrigeration needed)
Small can of tuna
Can of vegetarian low-fat chili
Luna bar (a healthy combination of carbohydrates and protein designed for women; Clif Bars are the men's counterpart)
Pretzels
Raw almonds

Perhaps you can think of other packaged treats you enjoy that will sustain you at emergency moments. A health food store is a good place to browse. Very often you can find items that aren't too processed but have lots of flavor.

Another strategy is to have in mind a meal that you can order automatically. For example, when I can't think of anything else to order and my blood sugar seems to be so low I feel like my power to reason has flown away, I automatically order a turkey sandwich on whole wheat with lettuce and tomato—light on the mayonnaise. That becomes my mantra when I can think of nothing else. It's very helpful, and it happens to be a sandwich you can get almost everywhere. Think about something you might like that's comparable.

Good sandwiches:

Sliced tomatoes on whole wheat toast with lettuce cut in shreds
This is my friend Rozanne Gold's favorite quick sandwich. She said the cut lettuce gives some bulk to the sandwich and the toast warms the tomatoes. She adds a slice of cheese. She is the author of Healthy 1-2-3.
Grilled vegetables in a wrap
The wrap phenomena may be waning a bit, but it's sure an easy way to eat and is so available. Try eating a salad in a wrap.
Soup (without cream base) and ½ sandwich

Avoid:

Tuna salad—too much mayonnaise
Quiche—made with many eggs and cheese
Creamy soups—contain too much fat
Caesar salad—dressing is very fatty, as are the croutons and the cheese sprinkled over the top.

Brunch

I personally love brunch. But it's such a challenge to be good. On weekends in New York City, the streets are filled with temptation: maple syrup is cascading off stacks of pancakes, melting cheese oozes from fluffy omelets, and giant muffins seem like they are out to get me. I wonder, do I count this as breakfast? Lunch? It all looks so good.

Let's slow down the temptation and come up with a game plan for brunch.

1. Don't go to brunch hungry. Have a light breakfast beforehand, such as a little yogurt and fruit or a very small portion of oatmeal.
2. Try to schedule brunch at lunchtime. You'll have many more menu choices that way. Brunch as breakfast means consuming a huge amount of carbs and fat.
3. Try to use this meal as a time to have fruit.
4. Many restaurants serve all-white omelets—made just with egg whites, this will help cut the fat out of the dish.
5. Order an omelet with lots of veggies in it.
6. Don't drink your meal! Skip the juice and eat fruit. It will fill you up more and take more time to consume.
7. Skip the complimentary cocktail. Many restaurants offer a champagne cocktail as part of a brunch—it's not worth it. Try a "virgin mary," a bloody mary without the vodka.

Buffets

A buffet does not mean you can strap on a feed bag. All of that food . . . and so many choices. It can be daunting. In a sense a buffet signals "all you can eat." Don't take it to heart (or back to your table). This is an opportunity to have a good time—with a little planning. Here are a few tips for coping with the abundance set before you:

- First, take one trip down the buffet line without a plate and get an overview of what's available. Think about the foods that you would really enjoy that fit into your plan.
- You don't have to be the first person in line. If you fill your

plate too fast and eat quickly, you'll be more tempted to go back again.

- Go for grains and beans, salads and veggies.
- Skip foods that look like they have a lot of cheese, mayonnaise, or heavy sauce.
- Be careful of salad dressings.
- Take one plate and don't go back for more.

Visiting Friends and Family

Some of the more pleasurable times in life are getting to spend time with friends and family, and visiting them at their homes. It's a warm and friendly environment, with people who have known you for years. But it can also be a minefield for sticking to your eating plan.

Picture this: You are visiting your cousin Lois for a family gathering. She serves Hawaiian chicken with pineapple. Do you

1. Eat it with gusto and figure you'll deal with your blood sugar tomorrow?
2. Ask if she has any chicken without the sauce?
3. Eat a little and pray for salad and vegetables?

Well, everyone might have a different answer. But the best method of dealing with situations like this is to actually develop a strategy before you get there.

It's best to expect the worst-case scenario when dining with friends or family. After all, they may have no idea of what your dietary needs are. So at the beginning of the day, anticipate this meal so that it can fit into your daily plan. Remember, no matter what—portion control! Keep in mind what your actual portion sizes are.

If you have found that all of the above fails and you eat more than you wanted and didn't stick with your eating plan, remember that it is only one meal. Try not to take this upset to your control personally. Even if you think Cousin Lois is insensitive to not think about your needs, it's not worth the argument now to try to make her realize this. Assume people want to do the right thing but don't always know what to do.

So do you alert your hosts about your dietary needs before you go to their house or should a visitor with diabetes just deal with what's being presented? I think this is a judgment call. Much depends on the event, the attitude of the hosts, and your relationship to them. Don't make a statement with your diabetes. Be gracious. If you eat only small portions of what is being served and skip entire courses, it's probably best to explain why. Often your hosts will be happy to include an extra large salad to the menu in consideration of your needs.

Special Events

At a dinner party one should eat wisely but not too well, and talk well but not too wisely.
—W. Somerset Maugham

Whether for our business or personal lives, there are events that we need to attend: weddings, parties, conferences, celebrations. For some, they are a weekly occurrence. For others, there may be only one or two a year. No matter how often, it takes some strategy to stay on track. This, like so many other aspects of diabetes, takes planning.

- Plan your eating schedule to accommodate the event.
- Work out before: you'll look better with a nice healthy glow and it will help curb your appetite.
- Drink a lot of water before and during the event. This will also decrease your appetite.
- Don't arrive hungry. Have a healthy snack before you go.
- Don't load up on hors d'oeuvres. The best strategy is to skip

the hors d'oeuvres entirely. It's easier to start by saying no and sticking to it than to lose your resolve bite by bite. If that's not possible, then try to go for the offerings that are vegetable based. Remember a dip may be fine, but if you're using chips, it's not! . . . Skip anything fried.

■ Limit alcohol. Drinking makes you forget your goals and uses up too many calories.

If you are at a sit-down dinner, you don't need to be a member of the Clean Plate Club: You don't have to eat and/or finish everything, especially items that aren't on your plan.

Special events can be stressful. Very often we feel on display and pressure to be on our best behavior, especially if the event is business related. This may be the wrong day to splurge, as it may upset your balance and make you feel bad about yourself afterward. Given the emotional charge that many special events are coupled with, I sometimes try to eat as little as possible at those occasions. Try putting your attention on the event itself rather than making the food the main attraction.

Holiday Survival Tips

Between Thanksgiving and New Year's is the black hole of all diets. Where did all the good intentions go? Where did my waistline go?

If you can, it's useful to prepare for the holidays as if you are training for a marathon. Try to rally before Halloween. If you miss that date, try as far before Thanksgiving as possible. Remember it's never too late to start anew. Stick to a healthy eating plan, exercise as much as you can, and get some extra rest. Any preparation will help give you more resolve during the holidays, compensate for some "slippage," and reduce stress, which can be in full force during busy times and lots of personal interactions.

Thanksgiving can be tricky because the very nature of the holiday is about abundance. If you are going to go overboard on anything, try sticking to the turkey and the plainest vegetable possible. The stuffing, cranberry jelly, and sweet potatoes can be overwhelming. See if you can arrange for a baked sweet potato instead of a "candied" preparation.

For holiday cocktail parties, try to follow the other suggestions in this chapter. Beware of egg nog. It's all cream and alcohol. Don't get started.

Traveling

No matter the distance or the time, travel requires extra management of your diabetes. Each form of travel can present different challenges. If traveling by air, you'll discover that many airlines have a diabetes meal. Be sure to order a special meal 48 hours in advance because most airlines have a cutoff. I personally have found "Diabetes Meals" to be just awful and do my best to bring my own nutritious food. Or, try the low-fat airline meal. Let the flight attendant know you have diabetes and need to keep your food consumption on schedule, and you might be able to get your meal in a timely fashion. Skip those nuts you are given with a beverage! Try to pack your own food when you can. No matter what, pack snacks in case you develop a low and the flight attendants aren't planning to serve at that moment.

Changing time zones can be a challenge for medication and insulin. Check with your doctor if you are on insulin so you can adjust it as you travel.

Tips for Food and Travel
By land, sea, or air:

- No matter what, check your glucose when you start your trip and frequently while traveling. When you arrive check again. It's sometimes hard to determine after the excitement of traveling if you have low blood sugar or jet lag.
- Have regular snacks to keep from having low blood sugar.
- Drink plenty of water. Plane travel can be dehydrating, so carry extra water with you.
- When traveling over time zones remember that traveling west

to east lengthens the day, which will increase your need for a snack. On the other hand, east to west shortens the day.

■ Try to walk a bit on the plane and, if you have time, at the airport.

When you arrive:

■ Have a food plan for your arrival. Do you have a restaurant already picked out and booked?

■ Look for menus posted in restaurant windows. Do they have several choices that fit into your plan?

■ When in foreign countries, carry a dictionary to restaurants in order to safeguard from choosing heavily sauced or sweetened food.

■ When sightseeing keep snacks and water with you at all times.

Sometimes dealing with the outside world feels daunting, especially when you first are developing a resolve to manage your diabetes. Don't give up and don't exclude all the special interactions you can have. It's more a question of emphasis. Put your attention on decor, ambience, or the true meaning of a special event. People gather for more than just to fill themselves up to the limit. Sometimes the excitement or tension inherent in being off our own turf can drop the safe cloak of determination. No matter what, as you venture forth, enjoy yourself and don't beat yourself up.

CHAPTER 10

Complementary Therapies for the Body, Mind, and Spirit

When you're at the doctor's office, it's easy to feel as though your whole life's experience and worth is reduced to a set of numbers examined: your blood glucose levels, triglycerides, and pounds of flesh. While these numbers are an invaluable guide to your doctor, they should not be the only things that you think about in terms of how you are coping with diabetes. Look at the whole picture of yourself—not just your weight or your glucose but your mind, body, and spirit. All are integrally related. If your body is feeling down, your mind and spirit will be feeling low as well. While your doctor seeks to take care of your body with her prescription of weight loss, exercise, medication, and tight control over your blood glucose, it is you who will carry out those recommendations. To do that effectively, you need to be responsible for the nourishment and health of your mind and spirit.

You are in charge of your own well-being. That is a scary concept to many people in this age of quick fixes and instant cures, but it is a concept that is certainly true to the management of diabetes. The best doctor in the world cannot force you to lose the weight you need to lose, or adjust your diet to keep your glucose levels in check, or exercise to keep your heart healthy. Doctors, nutritionists, and health practitioners are there to assist, but ultimately we all have to be responsible for ourselves.

Many of the lifestyle changes that are required in order to manage our diabetes require looking inside ourselves to examine our willingness or ability to make changes. For many of us it is a whole new experience. That is why it is important to know about complementary medicine when you are dealing with diabetes. This concept of healing takes the entire person into account and can be a useful aid in both self-discovery and overall good health. These alternative forms of medicine give us other avenues to explore in our quest to live well with diabetes, and will create another supportive team of people upon which we can rely and add to our circle of support.

The idea of complementary therapy, also known as alternative or integrative medicine, has been slowly gaining acceptance in the United States. For years, we have practiced what is called traditional "Western" medicine, but really, it is not traditional at all, as its practice has only come into fruition in the last 200 years or so. So what we call complementary, or alternative, medicine is actually the types of medicines that have been used for, in some cases, thousands of years in places such as China and India. In those countries it is "traditional" medicine, and is time-honored. Today, we in the West are just beginning to learn of its powerful effects on the body. The National Institutes of Health has opened a special department, called the National Center for Complementary and Alternative Medicine (NCCAM), that promotes exploration and research into these forms of medicinal therapies.

Over the years I have studied yoga, practiced meditation, and enjoyed many different forms of massage. But it is only since I was diagnosed with diabetes that I feel I have truly had an experience of the mind-body-spirit connection.

With the practice of alternative medicine, there seems to be a slower pace by healer and patient alike. These therapies require a closer look at each individual. The practitioner must include a view of the state of mind and spirit. And the modalities themselves take this into account as well. Unfortunately, mainstream medicine as controlled by managed care doesn't allow doctors to spend much time with each person they see. This results in a leveling of responses doctors can have. A diagnosis must be quick and the plan of action is equally universal. So it's particularly useful to explore alternative or complementary medicine as an adjunct to that experience. As you will see, some form of stress management, which has been shown can lower blood glucose levels, may be included.

In this chapter, we explore some of the alternative therapies that can have beneficial effects on people suffering from diabetes. But it is important to remember that complementary therapies do not replace what we have already discussed in treating diabetes: a healthy diet, exercise, visits with your doctor, medicine or insulin therapy if necessary, and regularly checking blood glucose levels. The reason we use the term *complementary* therapies, rather than *alternative,* is to emphasize the fact that these modes will complement your regular methods of living with diabetes.

Massage

There is nothing better than getting a massage, and to find out it is helpful with your diabetes is an added plus. Now you have a reason to indulge yourself, and you should think of massage not as a luxury but a necessity.

When you were born, you were held most of the day, and rocked, and nursed, and fed. As middle age comes upon us and seniority looms, it becomes more and more important to be touched, but it happens less and less often. As a society, we are "hands-off." Usually it's a quick handshake or a kiss on the cheek that you get—even from your dearest friends and relatives. Who among us wouldn't like their hands held for a little while each day?

Well, massage is one of the most healing of all touches. Massage has been found to provide some relief with many conditions. It is particularly useful for people with diabetes. It helps lower your blood pressure, improves circulation, reduces your heart rate, and sends out endorphins to your body for healing.

Massage's history is long. It has been traditionally used to promote healing for at least the last few thousand years in Rome, Persia, Greece, Japan, and Egypt, among others. Per Henrik Ling, a Swedish gymnast, revived its use in modern day and came up with many of the terms we use today for massage.

Massage can be done by yourself, by a loved one, or by a professional massage therapist. Just giving your feet a good massage at night can make a difference in circulation and overall well-being. Massage helps to circulate blood in your extremities, and blood circulation is a key element to healing. Tonight, try taking some lotion and gently massaging it on your feet. Gently give your toes a squeeze too. You will probably notice that if you do this for a little bit, your feet will be feeling warmer with the extra blood coming to your extremities, and your hands and feet will be smoother from the lotion.

Acupuncture

Acupuncture can be traced back thousands of years to China. It is based upon the idea that Qi (pronounced "chee") is the energy that flows through the body through meridians, which carry the energy to and from the body's essential systems. Administered by a certified acupuncturist, very small, thin needles are placed in meridians or energy points related to the area requiring attention for 20 to 30 minutes. Acupuncture is thought to maintain the harmonious flow of Qi, thus assuring good physical and mental health. There are many other traditional ways of maintaining good, healthy levels of Qi in the body, including healthy eating, breathing deeply of good, clean air, and exercise.

Next to nutrition therapy, acupuncture has been the most studied and perhaps admired of the alternative therapies from a Western perspective. The World Health Organization, the health branch of the United Nations, lists more than 40 conditions where acupuncture may be useful. Although diabetes is not included in this list, some of the symptoms of diabetes, such as pain, may be helped by acupuncture. Clinical studies have shown it to be an effective method for treating painful chronic peripheral neuropathy in diabetes. A group of patients underwent a 10-week course of six acupuncture treatments, and 77 percent of the patients found significant improvement in their pain; 67 percent were able to stop or reduce taking their drugs for the pain for a period of 52 weeks after the treatment ended (*Diabetes Research and Clinical Practice* 39, 2 [1998]: 115–21).

A National Institutes of Health panel in 1997 highlighted clinical studies indicating that acupuncture is an effective treatment for nausea incurred from surgical anesthesia, chemotherapy, and dental pain. It can also help with many different types of pain (headache, menstrual pain, fibromyalgia, arthritis, back pain), and may be useful with addiction and asthma and helping with stroke rehabilitation.

Some people are unnerved at the prospect of going to an acupuncturist because it sounds incredibly painful, having needles stuck in your body. But, while it may prove to be mildly uncomfortable for some, it is used to help with pain, not cause it. For many the insertion of the needles causes little to no pain. The needles used for acupuncture are extremely thin. Many people say that they feel a tingling sensation, which is supposed to be a good sign that Qi is arriving.

A health note: Make sure that all the needles used on you are brand new and for your use only. Complications are very rare, but may include infection, if the needles that are used are not sterile, and puncture of organs, if the needles are inserted too far.

Finding a good acupuncturist is very important. First, you can ask your doctor to see if she has any recommendations. As acupuncture becomes more and more validated as a useful medicinal tool, many doctors have found out more about the practice to help their patients. Ask friends and family for a reference. Also, contact your state health board and see who has been licensed in your area. Also refer to hospitals that may have alternative medicine as part of their makeup. It's likely that someone working with the hospital would be very reputable.

Relaxation Techniques

Meditation

In the '60s and '70s, when transcendental meditation was introduced to the United States, it was thought of as a practice for the very few. Now it has become quite mainstream. The effects can be significant. It is wonderful for stress management, can lower blood pressure, and can even have an effect on blood sugar levels. Meditation can take many forms, from repeating a "mantra" word or sentence or breath to merely observing one's thoughts.

I have found it is true that relaxation takes very little time (15 to 30 minutes) when compared to the results it produces during the day. It also seems to have a cumulative effect on your overall stress level. I've also found that when I feel stressed I can access the calming experience I have had when meditating and lower my agitation.

A simple way to meditate is just to spend a limited time with your eyes and body at rest and allow your mind to let go of much that seems significant. Another way to meditate by yourself is to use some of the many tapes in the library or bookstores that can lead you through a meditation. And the practice of yoga has a meditation component, so if you find a place that teaches yoga you will most likely find a way to learn meditation also.

Guided Imagery

This is a process that can lead to mental relaxation and healing. You are taken through a series of exercises that involve images, stories, and metaphors. According to Janelle D. White, M.D., an expert in herbal and preventative medicine, guided imagery may also be effective in lowering blood glucose levels.

Biofeedback

In biofeedback, blood pressure, temperature, heart rate, and other vital signs can be used to train yourself in techniques to calm yourself down and control bodily responses by altering brain activity. There are several types of biofeedback programs, but they all are meant to aid in relaxation for improvement of a variety of health problems. Positive results have been found in lowering glucose levels and pain due to neuropathy as well as blood pressure, anxiety, migraines, and sleep disorders. Most programs take 6 to 12 sessions, which then gives you the techniques for controlling these conditions yourself. You can find referrals at your local hospital.

Restorative Exercise

As emphasized throughout this book, exercise is essential for proper control of diabetes. You need to move, and there are many ways of going about it. Yoga and t'ai chi are two forms of exercise that have been practiced for thousands of years, yoga from India and t'ai chi from China. They promote balance, flexibility, and breath control.

Yoga

Yoga was developed in India more than two millennia ago. The Indians have the same viewpoint as the Chinese do about Qi—in their case the body's energy is called prana and flows through channels known as nadis. If all is flowing well in the body, it will remain healthy. But if prana is blocked, disease will result. The postures, breathing, and meditation in yoga were developed to remove the energy blockages in the body and mind. It is believed by the Hindus that, by controlling the body and calming the mind, it is possible to see the world and your place in it in its true light.

As yoga has been found to be so therapeutic, many hospitals now offer yoga classes as part of their community health projects, and yoga classes are held in most gyms. Most good yoga teachers have been extensively trained in their practice, with many having lived in India to study their craft. There are many different types of yoga practiced— some focus a lot on meditation, while others focus on warming up the body and building flexibility. Ask the yoga instructor about the kind of yoga practiced and the philosophies behind it. If you do take a class and find that it's either too active or too calm for you, discuss with your instructor other types of yoga that may suit your style more, and where those classes can be found.

Yoga is easy for anyone to start. You needn't feel pressured to try to attain all of the postures perfectly in your first few classes. It takes time and learning to get your body to that level of suppleness and flexibility, but anyone of any age should be able to participate in some form of yoga. (Please check with your doctor before embarking on any physical program.) Yoga is best done in loose, comfortable clothing, but not so loose that your instructor cannot see your body's lines in the posture. Also, yoga is normally done barefoot, so that you do not slip on the floor. Make sure you thoroughly check your feet after a yoga session to look for any damage to them, and check the floor around you before you start to make sure that the area around you is clean. It may be a good idea to discuss with your yoga teacher if there are any grippy, slipperlike shoes you can wear that would protect your feet and yet enable you to do the poses without slipping.

T'ai Chi

Perhaps we know t'ai chi from the pictures on television of the older people in China going through a series of slow exercises. Or perhaps you have a group in your hometown who practice together. Either way, t'ai chi is becoming a more and more popular form of gentle physical and mental exercise here in the West.

T'ai chi means "supreme ultimate" and refers to a system of exercise and breathing that seeks to improve the energy, or chi (Qi), in your body. T'ai chi comes from very ancient practices, but has been further developed over the last two centuries in China. It's move to the West has really come in the last 20 years or so, as we explore alternate forms of thought and exercise. Certainly one of the most intriguing aspects of this exercise is that it can be practiced well into old age and keeps your golden years as active and supple as possible. It improves respiration for the heart and lungs, and calms the mind. Seek out t'ai chi classes at your local gym, health center, or adult education program. There are also many wonderful videos out there for you to follow in the comfort of your own home.

Nutrition Therapy

Nutrition therapy is the cornerstone of living with diabetes (see chapter 4). For diabetes, nutrition therapy is a healthy diet that spreads carbohydrates evenly throughout the day, is reduced in fats (especially saturated fats), high in fiber, and provides adequate amounts of protein, vitamins, minerals, water, and calories.

In addition to a healthy diet and active lifestyle, some health care professionals recommend using herbs and dietary supplements to help lower blood glucose levels or treat diabetic complications.

Commonly used herbs include:

- Grape seed extract—it may have antioxidant properties.
- Fenugreek seeds and seed extract—it may lower blood glucose levels.
- Gymnema sylvestre—it may lower blood glucose levels.
- Aloe vera—used externally aloe vera may enhance healing of wounds, and used internally it may lower blood glucose and triglyceride levels.
- Garlic—either fresh or from commercially produced tablets, garlic may help with hypertension and lowering elevated cholesterol levels. However, garlic may cause an unpleasant taste and bad breath, heartburn, flatulence, and other gastrointestinal discomfort. People taking aspirin or any other anticoagulant medications should avoid taking large dosages of garlic.

Commonly used vitamins include:

- Vitamin E—it may act as an antioxidant.
- Vitamin C—it may act as an antioxidant.
- B vitamins (including B_6, B_{12}, folic acid, and biotin).

Some commonly used minerals include:

- Chromium
- Magnesium

Although the jury may be out on the benefits of certain herbal supplements, there are other reasons to take special care if you are planning surgery. Researchers at the University of Indiana have warned that certain herbal supplements may contribute to complications during surgery. It is important to let your doctor know what supplements you are taking even if they are the over-the-counter variety, and it's wise to stop certain types two weeks before an operation.

Although supplementing a healthy meal plan with dietary supplements and herbs may be helpful in treating diabetes, you should be very cautious when doing so. Some herbs or supplements may have adverse interactions with medications. Be sure to consult your physician or health care provider before taking any herbal or dietary supplement, especially if you are taking any medications.

Possible drug-herb/supplement interactions:

Glipizide—magnesium hydroxide, fenugreek, and Gymnema sylvestre
Glyburide—chromium, biotin, vitamin E, aloe vera, and Gymnema sylvestre

This chapter should have given you some ideas of what is available beyond traditional medicine, and it is by no means comprehensive. These forms of healing have their roots in ancient traditions, but they can address modern problems. When you participate in this type of healing modality, you are saying to yourself that all your individual needs—from your spirit to your mind to your body—can be taken into account. Coupled with modern medicine, you can approach taking care of yourself for a lifetime.

CHAPTER 11

Pampering as Medicine

Exercise! Watch what you eat! Check your glucose levels! There's so much to do when you've got diabetes. Hopefully you now understand the importance of these activities, and at some point during the reading of this book you have begun to incorporate them into your daily activities. If you have, bravo. And if so, you can use this chapter as a way of exploring other aspects of care. If you have been recently diagnosed or you have had difficulty in integrating your diabetes management into your life, I hope this chapter assists you in looking inside yourself to make changes.

Real Possibilities

As we care for our bodies it's important to know that we can never really separate our bodies from our mind and spirit. In order to take the best care of ourselves over time, we need to be mindful inside and out. The message of this chapter is that medicine comes in many forms. When we are good to ourselves we are providing important healing for our entire being. Pampering as medicine can involve anything from taking a little time to do the things you love to going to a spa for delicious time to concentrate on yourself. First some food for thought and then some ideas of ways to treat yourself.

Diabetes has such a strong impact on everything we do. So much so that even if we are in denial about the disease we are still involved with it. It still affects our lives. In other words, even if we try to ignore it we are still reacting to it either actively or passively. We always have a choice about how we want to deal with it. Do we want to take it head-on, sweep it under the carpet, educate ourselves, or try to avoid the issues?

Often people tell me that it's great that I have made "lemonade out of lemons." That may appear to be what I have done, but more than any action I've taken, I have had to come up against my own point of view about myself. There have been so many times over these years that I have said to myself, "It doesn't matter what I do" or "What difference does it make?" I live alone and frequently I ask, "Who cares what I do?"

Because diabetes requires so much self-care and self-management, it requires us to come to grips with our own self-worth, because if we don't place a premium on our own lives, how can we do the many things required? One way or another, we are forced to ask ourselves: How much do we truly value ourselves and what actions do we take in order to communicate that to ourselves? If a loved one sent us flowers or planned a special night out, wouldn't we say to ourselves that they really cared about us?

What messages do we send to ourselves? Do the ripped pajamas give us sweet dreams? Does eating out of the refrigerator make us feel special? Every act has a subtle and sometimes not so subtle effect on our own point of view about ourselves.

Often we look outside ourselves for our own worth. If someone praises us we feel good. We get a job promotion—we're brilliant. We lose a job—we are worthless. We are honored in our community—we are honorable people. These are all external cues. But what do we truly feel about ourselves? I'd like to suggest that diabetes gives us an opportunity to examine how we value ourselves on the deepest level—and to fight for ourselves too.

If my son, Noah, needed care I would do anything in my power to make sure he had what he needed. There isn't a day that goes by that I'm not involved with my mother's well-being. Do I treat myself with the same fierce commitment? Am I willing to go the limit for myself? I wish I could turn my diabetes management over to someone else, but I know after these years with diabetes that I must dig down and find the commitment to myself that I show to my loved ones.

Why is being good to yourself a special occasion?

Of course, among other things, we all need to watch what we are eating, exercise, check our blood sugar, and, for most, take medication. But why are some of us ready to charge ahead with our own care while others are not? Whatever age we are, this is the time to make your own health and well-being a top priority.

 Ask Yourself

If you say that you don't have time in your schedule to exercise or take time for yourself, look to see where you have placed yourself on a list of your top priorities. Have you trained yourself and those around you that you do not come first? Ever? Hardly ever? Only on special occasions? And why would being good to yourself have to be a special occasion? Doesn't that say something?

Pampering not only communicates internally that you care about yourself, it also creates an atmosphere of well-being for those around you. Whether acknowledged in a family or not, illness, depression, and lack of buoyancy dampens those attached to you. Have you had loved ones who weren't taking appropriate care of themselves? What does that do to your sense of joy in living? So if you have difficulty with the concept of simply putting yourself on an upper rung of life's ladder, think about the effect of your well-being on others.

Ideas for Pampering

Each one of us has to decide what signals special treatment. For some, a few hours of quiet time away from the demands of the family may be a little bit of heaven, while for others a trip to a spa signals that pampering is in progress (I can't imagine that's not so for most folks). Yet pampering is more about attitude than expense. It's about you finding your special treatment. In any case, here are some suggestions ranging from the simple to the sublime.

Deluxe Pampering

There are a number of excellent spas or health resorts in the United States. Some emphasize fitness, others, like the Green Door spas, concentrate more on pampering. Some, like Canyon Ranch Health Resorts, provide the full range of experiences from vigorous athletics to spiritual awareness. Canyon Ranch resorts have a special separate nurturing environment on the grounds called the Life Enhancement Center, where people can deal in depth with specific health issues. Other spas and health centers have special weeks for people with diabetes, including the Hilton Head Health Resort in Hilton Head Island, South Carolina. Watch for notices at your local diabetes center for other spa/health resorts that have time devoted to diabetes care.

Even if there isn't a special week devoted to diabetes, it's so beneficial to take time in an environment that supports health and well-being. Look at a publication called *Spa Finders* for further information.

Sometimes even getting away overnight can be a way of nurturing yourself. Many hotels have special weekend rates. A dear friend uses this as an opportunity to say good-bye to her husband and two-year-old for a night of room service, a hot bath, and uninterrupted sleep.

As a New Yorker, removing myself from an urban environment for a day or two becomes a necessity. When I can't go far, I cross over to New Jersey, where I've found a few hotels that have built-in spas. An overnight stay and a walk through a little greenery is a quick and pampering adventure.

Check with your local travel agent for cruise ships that now provide special spa services and guest lecturers on health and nutrition.

Pampering for Less

Does getting away in this fashion seem as realistic as a trip to the Emerald City? Many communities have day spas that create a setting that will "take you away" for a few hours. An alternative is to join with a few friends and create a day spa at home. Join forces and hire a personal trainer for a group. Ask a local manicurist to come in for some treatments or buy the supplies and take care of one another.

Is there a sport that you have always wanted to do? Perhaps a few lessons will set you on the right track.

My friend Margo and I go to a local storefront where you can decorate pre-molded pottery. We feel like school kids again as we paint with aprons on as the shop assistant encourages us with new painting techniques. We are currently making plates with our handprints for our grown-up sons.

Making breakfast, lunch, and dinner every night for some is a real chore. For many, a special meal in an elegant restaurant may be just the ticket for taking great care of yourself. Here is another point of view:

From the time I was a young adult, I loved to cook and then, about five years ago, slowly got out of the habit. I ran a program at NYU that taught nutrition students the importance of proper food preparation, but by the time I got home, my own cooking was the last thing I wanted to do. Pots and pans and sharpened knives stood waiting at attention while slowly, one dinner after another, I turned over meal preparation to restaurants and ordering in.

Because many of my friends are in the food business, as I was years ago, I have many opportunities to try new restaurants and attend food-related events. Seems like a dream—New York City, parties, food adventures. What could be missing? How about a sense of nurturing myself? I began to feel like I was consuming food (usually quite healthy and balanced) but I wasn't using this as special time for myself. I have rediscovered the importance of cooking for myself. I did it first by changing my thinking about it. Rather than a nuisance at the end of the day, I started to think about the message I sent to myself when I cooked. I began to use shopping for fresh food and the preparation as a way of being good to myself. This was my special time. Choosing fresh and pleasing produce became another way to pamper myself. I was buying this for me! I made friends with the fish man. Visits to the local greenmarket connected me to the farmers who grew the food I was taking home. The time I spent peeling and chopping became a way to put aside the day and return to a more quiet joy. I also found that I naturally lost some more weight. I was in control of the ingredients. So the whole process has become a way to pamper myself.

> Because he was dining alone, his cook assumed a simple meal would do, but his error was quickly corrected when Lucullus responded, "What? Did you not know, then, that today Lucullus dines with Lucullus?"   —Plutarch

So whatever you choose, ultimately, pampering is a state of mind. It's the willingness to take a deep breath and remember or discover who you really are. This is where real discovery comes from. You can go do all of the many things you are told to do. But healing begins within. Invest in your spirit. When you do you will be able to look at real life, as complicated and messy as it can be, with a sense of new real possibilities.

appendixes

Sample Menus

Chapter 4 presented eating plans and some basic nutritional advice, including three different levels of eating based on your glucose levels, from simple adjustments to a more detailed system, the diabetic exchange system. Whatever way you choose to eat in a healthy manner, these menus will give you a sense of how one can eat a balanced and varied diet on any given day. The portions are listed to indicate appropriate amounts and encourage moderation without excessive restriction. Note that the protein, fats, and carbohydrates are spread throughout the day to help maintain energy and avoid spikes in glucose levels. To count the number of carbohydrates servings, add starch, fruit, and dairy. This is based on an 1,800-calorie plan.

Level 1

Menu A

Breakfast
1 cup whole-grain cereal
¼ sliced banana and ½ cup fresh blueberries
1 cup fat-free milk
1 cup V8 juice

Lunch

Chicken fajita with whole-grain wrap (including 3 ounces chicken, green and yellow peppers, sautéed onions, corn, and red pepper)

Jicama salad with tomato vinaigrette

Afternoon snack

2 tablespoons scallion hummus with whole-grain pita and baby carrots

Dinner

1 slice turkey meatloaf

½ cup barley pilaf

Brussels sprouts and walnuts

Watercress, mushroom, and endive salad with balsamic vinaigrette

Bedtime snack

1 medium baked apple with low-fat creamy topping

Servings, Level 1, Menu A

	Grain/ Starch	Vegetable	Fruit	Protein	Dairy	Fat
Breakfast	2	unlimited	1		1	
Lunch	2	unlimited		3		1
Snack	2	unlimited				
Dinner	1	unlimited		4–5		2
Snack			1		1	

Menu B

Breakfast

Kiwi-strawberry shake made with ½ cup fruit and 1 cup fat-free milk

¼ cup scrambled egg substitute with spinach

Lunch

Bean burritos (made with ¼ cup beans and 1 ounce low-fat cheese, avocado, lettuce, and tomato)

½ cup rice with onions

Shredded carrot salad

Afternoon snack

⅓ cup raw almonds

1 small apple, sliced

Dinner

5 ounces broiled salmon with tomatoes and olives

1 cup whole-wheat couscous with pine nuts and currants

Cucumber and dill salad

Bedtime snack

2 graham crackers

1 tablespoon peanut butter

Servings, Level 1, Menu B

	Grain/ Starch	Vegetable	Fruit	Protein	Dairy	Fat
Breakfast		unlimited	1	1	1	1
Lunch	3	unlimited	1		1	2
Snack			1		1	
Dinner	2	unlimited		5		
Snack	1				½	

Level 2

Menu A

Breakfast

¼ cup low-fat granola with 1 cup nonfat plain yogurt topped with 2 tablespoons raisins

Lunch

Tuna Niçoise salad with dill vinaigrette

(including 3½-ounce can tuna, 2 small red potatoes, string beans, capers, and romaine lettuce)

Afternoon snack

2 or 3 whole-grain crackers

2 tablespoons chive tofu spread

Dinner

Grilled red snapper

Roasted fennel

Polenta with 1 ounce goat cheese

Sautéed kale

Bedtime snack

1 cup of sliced strawberries with fat-free whipped topping

Servings, Level 2, Menu A

	Grain/ Starch	Vegetable	Fruit	Protein	Dairy	Fat
Breakfast	2		1		1	
Lunch	2	unlimited		3.5		1
Snack	1			1		
Dinner	2	unlimited		5	1	2
Snack			1			

Menu B

Breakfast

2–egg white omelet filled with 1 ounce smoked salmon and 1 tablespoon fat-free cream cheese

1 whole-grain English muffin

1 small orange

Lunch

Chicken stir-fry with 3 ounces chicken and napa cabbage, red bell peppers, broccoli, bok choy, and fresh ginger

1 cup brown rice

Afternoon snack

½ cup lentil soup

Dinner

4 ounces marinated flank steak

1 cup quinoa topped with chopped walnuts

Green beans

Stewed tomatoes

Nighttime snack

Smoothie made with 1 cup nonfat milk, 1 cup strawberries, and mango

Servings, Level 2, Menu B

	Grain/ Starch	Vegetable	Fruit	Protein	Dairy	Fat
Breakfast	2		1	1	1	1
Lunch	2	unlimited		3		1
Snack	1					
Dinner	2	unlimited		4		2
Snack			1		1	

Level 3

Menu A

Breakfast
Frittata made with 2 eggs, sautéed onion, basil, and tomato
1 cup yams

Lunch
Mixed vegetable and turkey pita pocket with 2 ounces turkey and radishes, zucchini, sliced red onions, lettuce, and 2 tablespoons hummus

Cucumber, scallion, and romaine salad with mint yogurt dressing

Afternoon snack
¼ cup muesli
1 cup fat-free milk
½ banana

Dinner
4-ounce sautéed veal cutlet on a bed of Swiss chard
Zucchini, mushrooms, tomatoes, and garlic
½ cup white beans and sage

Nighttime snack
1 cup nonfat plain yogurt flavored with vanilla and strawberry puree topped with 1 ounce multigrain cereal

Servings, Level 3, Menu A

	Grain/ Starch	Vegetable	Fruit	Protein	Dairy	Fat
Breakfast	2	unlimited		2		1
Lunch	2	unlimited		2		1
Snack	1		1		1	
Dinner	1	unlimited		4		1
Snack	1		1		1	

Menu B

Breakfast

Strawberry and banana tofu shake (made with 4 ounces tofu and 1 cup fruit)

1 cup oatmeal

Lunch

Roasted chicken salad with red pepper puree dressing

(includes 3 ounces chicken, steamed asparagus, cherry tomatoes, ½ cup corn)

Afternoon Snack

½ cup melon

1 cup nonfat yogurt

¼ cup fiber cereal

Dinner

Lamb shish kebab with rosemary (made with 4 ounces lamb)

1 cup bulgar wheat

Roasted eggplant with garlic

Nighttime snack

¼ cup low-fat cottage cheese

3 pieces whole-grain melba toast

Servings, Level 3, Menu B

	Grain/ Starch	Vegetable	Fruit	Protein	Dairy	Fat
Breakfast	2		1	1		
Lunch	1	unlimited		3		1
Snack	1		1		1	
Dinner	2	unlimited		4		2
Snack	1				1	

Resources

Information Via Mail and Telephone

American Amputee Foundation
P.O. Box 250218
Little Rock, AR 72225
Phone: (501) 666-2523

American Association of Diabetes Educators
100 West Monroe Street
4th floor
Chicago, IL 60603
Phone: (800) 338-3633
www.aadcnet.org

American Board of Medical Specialties
1007 Church Street, Suite 404
Evanston, IL 60201
Phone: (866) ASK-ABMS

American Board of Podiatric Surgery
3330 Mission Street
San Francisco, CA 94100
Phone: (415) 826-3200
www.abps.org

American Council of the Blind
1155 15th Street NW, Suite 1004

Washington, DC 20005
Phone: (800) 424-8666
www.acb.org

American Dietetic Association
Headquarters/Chicago Office
216 West Jackson Boulevard, Suite 800
Chicago, IL 60606
Phone: (312) 899-0040; (800) 366-1655
www.eatright.org

American Dietetic Association
Washington, D.C., Office
1120 Connecticut Avenue NW, Suite 480
Washington, DC 20036
Phone: (202) 775-8277

American Heart Association
National Headquarters
7272 Greenville Avenue
Dallas, TX 75231
Phone: (800) 242-8721
www.americanheart.org

American Medical Association
515 North State Street
Chicago, IL 60610
Phone: (312) 464-4818
www.ama-assn.org

Canadian Diabetes Association
National Office
15 Toronto Street, Suite 800
Toronto, Ontario M5C 2E3
CANADA

Phone: (800) BANTING (from Canada only)
www.diabetes.ca

Diabetes Division
Centers for Disease Control and Prevention
National Center for Chronic Disease Prevention and Health
Promotion
TISB Mail Stop K-10
4770 Buford Highway NE
Atlanta, GA 30341
Phone: (877) CDC-DIAB
www.cdc.gov/diabetes

Diabetes Exercise and Sports Association (DESA)
P.O. Box 1935
Litchfield Park, AZ 85340
Phone: (800) 898-4322 or
(623) 535-4593
www.diabetes-exercise.org

The Diabetes Research and Wellness Foundation
1206 Potomac Street NW
Washington, DC 20007
Phone: (202) 298-9211
    or

The Diabetes Research and Wellness Center
189 Bradley Place
Palm Beach, FL 33480
Phone: (561) 802-3600
  or toll-free (877) 633-3976
www.diabeteswellness.org

Diabetic Retinopathy Foundation
350 North La Salle Street, Suite 800

Chicago, IL 60610
www.retinopathy.org

International Diabetes Federation (IDF)
Executive Office
1, rue Defacqz
B-1000 Brussels
BELGIUM
Phone: 32-21538 5511
www.idf.org

Joslin Diabetes Center
1 Joslin Place
Boston, MA 02215
Phone: (800) JOSLIN1
www.joslin.org

Medic Alert Foundation
2323 Colorado Avenue
Turlock, CA 95382
Phone: (800) 432-5378
www.medicalert.org

National Amputation Foundation
3840 Church Street
Malverne, NY 11565
Phone: (516) 887-3600
www.nationalamputation.org

National Diabetes Information Clearinghouse
1 Information Way
Bethesda, MD 20892
Phone: (800) 860-8747
or (301) 468-2162
www.niddk.nih.gov

National Federation for the Blind
1800 Johnson Street
Baltimore, MD 21230
Phone: (410) 659-9314
www.nfb.org/diabetes.htm

National Kidney Foundation
30 East 33rd Street
New York, NY 10016
Phone: (800) 622-9010
www.kidney.org

Wound Care Institute, Inc.
1100 N.E. 163rd Street, Suite 101
North Miami Beach, FL 33162
Phone: (305) 919-9192
www.woundcare.org

Journals and Magazines

Diabetes Advocate
American Diabetes Association
Government Relations Department
1660 Duke Street
Alexandria, VA 22314
Phone: (800) 342-2383

Diabetes Forecast
American Diabetes Association
1660 Duke Street
Alexandria, VA 22314
Phone: (800) 342-2383

Diabetes Self-Management
R.A. Rapaport Publishing, Inc.
150 West 22nd Street

New York, NY 10011
Phone: (800) 234-0923

Prevention
Customer Service
P.O. Box 7319
Red Oak, IA 51591
Phone: (800) 813-8070
www.healthyideas.com

Journals
British Medical Journal
BMJ Publishing Group
P.O. Box 590A
Kennebunkport, MA 04046
Phone: (800) 236-6265
www.bmj.com/bmj

Harvard Health Letter
Harvard University Publications
164 Longwood Avenue
Boston, MA 02115
Phone: (617) 432-1485
www.countwaymed.harvard.edu/publications/Health

Integrative Medicine
Elsevier Science
P.O. Box 945
New York, NY 10159
Phone: (888) 437-4636

Toll-Free Hotlines
American Dietetic Association and National Center for Nutrition and Dietetics (NCND) (800) 366-1655

American Podiatric Medical Association: (800) FOOTCARE

Pharmaceutical Company Customer Care Lines
Bayer Diagnostics Division: (800) 348-8100

Boehringer Mannheim Corporation: (800) 858-8072

Cascade Medical: (800) 525-6718

Lifescan, a Johnson & Johnson company: (800) 227-8862

Medisense, Inc.: (800) 527-3339

Websites
General Sites
Alternative treatments: www.alternativediabetes.com

American Diabetes Association: www.diabetes.org

American Massage Therapy Association: www.amtamassage.org

British Diabetes Association: www.diabetes.org.uk

Canadian Diabetes Association: www.diabetes.ca

Centers for Disease Control and Prevention (CDC):
www.cdc.gov or www.cdc.gov/diabetes

Diabetes self-management: www.diabetes-self-mgmt.com

Doctor's Guide to the Internet—Diabetes: www.docguide.com

General information from endocrinologists: www.endocrinolo-
gist.com/diabetes.htm

The Healing Handbook for Persons with Diabetes:
www.umassmed.edu/diabeteshandbook

International Diabetes Federation: www.idf.org

Joslin Diabetes Center: www.joslin.org

Managing your diabetes: www.lillydiabetes.com

National Center for Complementary and Alternative Medicine: www.nccam.nih.gov

National Diabetes Education Program: www.ndep.nih.gov

National Institute of Diabetes and Digestive and Kidney Diseases (NIDDK): www.niddk.nih.gov

National Institute on Aging: www.nih.gov/nia

Complications

American Cancer Society: www.cancer.org

American Heart Association: www.americanheart.org

American Institute for Cancer Research: www.aicr.org

Amputation Prevention Global Research Center: www.diabetes-resource.com

Heart Information Network: www.heartinfo.org

Mayo Health Clinic: www.mayohealth.org

National Eye Institute: www.nei.nih.gov

National Federation of the Blind: www.nfb.org/diabetes.htm

National Heart, Lung, and Blood Institute: www.nhlbi.nih.gov/index.htm

National Stroke Association: www.stroke.org

Wound care: www.woundcare.org

Race and Diabetes

American Diabetes Association's African-American Program: www.diabetes.org/africanamerican

Diabetes in African Americans: www.niddk.nih.gov/health/diabetes/pubs/afam/afam.htm

Diabetes in Hispanic Americans: www.niddk.nih.gov/health/diabetes/pubs/hispan/hispan.htm

Información para personas con diabetes: www.cica.es

"The Pima Indians: Pathfinders for Health": www.niddk.nih.gov/health/diabetes/pima/index.htm

Nutrition

American Dietetic Association: www.eatright.org

American Society for Nutritional Sciences: www.nutrition.org

Calories in food and beverages: www.nal.usda.gov/fnic/foodcomp

Food and Drug Administration: www.fda.gov

FDA information about dietary supplements: vm.cfsan.fda.gov/~dms/supplmnt.html

Health Canada: www.hc-sc.gc.ca

The International Food Information Council: www.ificinfo.health.org/index2-4.htm

Mayo Clinic Nutrition Center: www.mayohealth.org/mayo

Thrive Online: www.thriveonline.com

The Tufts University Nutrition Navigator: www.navigator.
tufts.edu

USDA dietary guidelines: www.nal.usda.gov/fnic/dga

USDA Food Guide Pyramid: www.nalusda.govworks

USDA search: www.usda.gov/search/index.htm

U.S. Government Healthfinder: www.healthfinder.gov

Exercise

AMA Health Insight's Fitness Basics: www.ama-assn.org

American College of Sports Medicine: www.acsm.org

Diabetes Exercise and Sports Association: www.diabetes-
exercise.org

Shape Up America: www.shapeup.org/sua

Surgeon general's report on physical activity: www.cdc.gov/
nccdphp/sgr/sgr.htm

Alternative Therapies

Alternative therapies for diabetes: www.niddk.nih.gov/health/
diabetes/summary/altmed/altmed.htm

"Medicine, Magic and Mumbo Jumbo": www.diabetes-self-
mgmt.com/index.php?page-ma97art

National Center for Complementary and Alternative Medicine: nccam.nih.gov

Travel

Nutrition for Diabetes: Eating Tips for Travelers: www.med.umich.edu/ilibr/topics/diabet10.htm

Money

Financial help for diabetes care: www.niddk.nih.gov/health/ diabetes/summary/finanass/finanass.htm

Diabetes Books

The Diabetes Mall: www.diabetesnet.com

Bibliography

Alper, Joe. "New Insight into Type 2 Diabetes." *Science* 289 (2000): 37–39.

American Diabetes Association. *Annual Review of Diabetes 2000*. Alexandria, Va.: American Diabetes Association, Inc., 2000.

———. *Complete Guide to Diabetes*. 2nd ed. Alexandria: American Diabetes Association, Inc., 1999.

———. *Diabetes 2001 Vital Statistics*. Alexandria: American Diabetes Association, Inc., 2001.

———. *Diabetes A to Z*. 3rd ed. Alexandria: American Diabetes Association, Inc., 1997.

———. *Medical Management of Type 2 Diabetes*. 4th ed. Alexandria, Va.: American Diabetes Association, Inc., 1998.

———. "Type 2 Diabetes in Children and Adolescents." *Diabetes Care* 23, 3 (2000): 381; 10.

American Diabetes Association/American Dietetic Association. *Exchange Lists for Meal Planning*. Alexandria: American Diabetes Association, Inc., 1995.

Anderson, Bob, and Martha Funnell. *The Art of Empowerment*. Alexandria, Va.: American Diabetes Association, Inc., 2000.

aofas.org. "Diabetic Foot." American Orthopaedic Foot and Ankle Society. http://www.aofas.org/diabeticfoot.asp

Bell, David S. H. "Alcohol and the NIDDM Patient." *Diabetes Care* 19, 5 (1996): 509–11.

Bernstein, Gerald. "Type 2 Diabetes in Children and Adolescents." *Practical Diabetology* Sept. 2000: 37–41.

Bjerkness, Sandy, and Greg Hagen. "Switching from Animal to Human Insulin." *Diabetes Self-Management* Mar.-Apr. 2001: 70–75.

Brand-Miller, Janette, et al. "Diets with a Low Glycemic Index: From Theory to Practice." *Nutrition Today* 34, 2 (1999): 64–98.

Brand-Miller, Jennie, et al. *The Glucose Revolution*. New York: Marlowe and Company, 1999.

Braunwald, Eugene, et al., eds. *Harrison's Principles of Internal Medicine*. 15th ed. New York: McGraw and Hill, 2001.

Cardiology.com. "Insulin Therapy a Predictor of Mortality in Coronary Artery Disease." Reuters Medical News. Apr. 2, 2001.

Castelli, William P., and Glen C. Griffin. *The New Good Fat Bad Fat*. Tucson, Ariz.: Fisher Books, 1997.

Castleman, Michael. "Men, Sex & Diabetes," April 2000. Diabetes.com

Chandalia, Manisha, et al. "Beneficial Effects of High Dietary Fiber Intake in Patients with Type 2 Diabetes Mellitus." *The New England Journal of Medicine* 342, 19 (2000): 1392–441.

Clark, C. M., et al. "Gestational Diabetes: Should It Be Added to the Syndrome of Insulin Resistance?" *Diabetes Care* 20, 5 (1997): 867–71.

Collins, Geneva. "Diabetes: Take it Seriously." *The Female Patient*. Chatham, N.J.: Quadrant Publishing, 1997.

Consumers Union. "Do You Know Your Blood-Sugar Level?" *Consumer Reports on Health* 12, 7 (2000): 1–5.

D'Arrigo, Terri. "Diabetes Pills and Gestational Diabetes." *Diabetes Forecast* May 2001: 106.

De Lorenzo, A., et al. "New Insights into Body Composition Assessment in Obese Women." *Canadian Journal of Physiology and Pharmacology* 77, 1 (1999): 17–21.

De Lucio-Brock, Jeff. "The Glycemic Index." Online posting. Updated April 2000. 14 Mar. 2001.

The Diabetes Control and Complications Trial Research Group. "The Effect of Intensive Treatment of Diabetes on the Development and Progression of Long-Term Complications in Insulin-Dependent Diabetes Mellitus." *The New England Journal of Medicine* 329, 14 (1993): 977–86.

Diabetes Forecast: Women & Diabetes. Alexandria, Va.: American Diabetes Association, Inc., May 2001.

diabetes.org. "African American Program." http://www.diabetes.org/main/community/outreach/african_americans/default.jsp

diabetes.org. "Eye Care and Retinopathy: Early Detection and Treatment of Eye Problems Can Save Your Sight." American Diabetes Association. http://www.diabetes.org/main/application/commercewf?origin=*.jsp&event=link(D3_3)

diabetes.org. "Gum Disease." American Diabetes Association. http://www.diabetes.org/main/application/commercewf?origin=navigation.jsp&event=link(C3_2)

diabetes.org. "Women's Sexual Health." diabetes.org/main/application/commercewf?origin=*.jsp&event=link(D2_4a)

diabetesincontrol.com. "TV Can Cause Diabetes in Young?" *BMJ* 2001; 322:313–314. diabetesincontrol.com/issue39/item7.htm

Diabeteswell.com. "Diabetes Snack Bars: Hype or Help?" 16 Mar. 2001 <http://www.diabeteswell.com/education/nutrition/snackbar.asp>.

Diabeticdiet.com. "Diabetes Snack Bars and Drinks: To Buy or Leave on the Shelf?" 16 Mar. 2001 <http://www.diabeticdiet.com/dd_nutrition1.htm>.

Edelwich, Jerry, and Archie Brodsky. *Diabetes: Caring for Your Emotions as well as Your Health.* Reading, Pa.: Perseus Books, 1998.

El-Rufaie, O. E. "Sexual Dysfunction among Type II Diabetic Men: A Controlled Study." *Journal of Psychosomatic Research* 43, 6 (1997): 605–12.

Familydoctor.org. "Exercise and Diabetes." 10 Mar. 2001 <http://www.familydoctor.org/handouts/351.html>.

Ferriss, Frederick L., et al. "Treatment of Diabetic Retinopathy." *The New England Journal of Medicine* 341, 9 (1999): 667–78.

Feskens, Edith J. M., J. Gerard Loeber, and Daan Kromhout. "Diet and Physical Activity as Determinants of Hyperinsulinemia: The Zutphen Elderly Study." *Journal of Epidemiology* 140, 4 (1994): 350–60.

The First Step in Diabetes Meal Planning. Alexandria, Va.: American Diabetes Association and American Dietetic Association, 1997.

Fletcher, Anne M. *Thin for Life.* Shelburne, Vt.: Chapters, 1994.

Formanek, Raymond. "FDA Approves Watch-like Device to Monitor Blood Sugar Levels." *FDA Consumer,* May-June, 2001: 7.

Franz, Marion J. "Exercise and the Management of Diabetes Mellitus." *Journal of the American Dietetic Association* 87, 7 (1987): 872–82.

Franz, Marion J., and John P. Bantle, eds. *American Diabetes Association Guide to Medical Nutrition Therapy for Diabetes.* Alexandria: American Diabetes Association, Inc., 1999.

Fritsch, Jane. "Scientists Unmask Diet Myth: Willpower." Nytimes.com 6 Oct. 1999 <http://www.nytimes.com/library.nati.../100599hth-nutritionwillpower.html>.

Fukagawa, Naomi K., et al. "High-Carbohydrate, High-Fiber Diets Increase Peripheral Insulin Sensitivity in Health Young and Old Adults." *American Journal of Clinical Nutrition* 52 (1990): 524–28.

Gaball, L. L., D. Godman-Gruen, and E. Barret-Connor. "The Effect of Postmenopausal Estrogen Therapy on the Risk of Non-Insulin-Dependent Diabetes Mellitus." *American Journal of Public Health* 87(3):443–5, March 1997.

Giller, Robert M., and Kathy Matthews. *Natural Prescriptions.* New York: Ballantine, 1994.

Groff, James L., Sareen S. Gropper, and Sara M. Hunt. *Advanced Nutrition and Human Metabolism.* 2nd ed. St. Paul, Minn.: West Publishing Company, 1995.

Grundy, Scott M., et al. "Diabetes and Cardiovascular Disease." *Circulation* 100 (1999): 1134–46.

Gu, Ken, et al. "Diabetes and Decline in Heart Disease Mortality in US Adults." *Journal of the American Medical Association* 281, 14 (1999): 1291–97.

Guthrie, Diana W. *Alternative and Complementary Diabetes Care.* New York: John Wiley & Sons, Inc., 2000.

Hagander, Barbro, et al. "Dietary Fiber Decreases Fasting Blood Glucose Levels and Plasma LDL Concentration in Non-Insulin-Dependent Diabetes Mellitus Patients." *American Journal of Clinical Nutrition* 47 (1988): 852–58.

Hansen, Barbara Caleen, and Shauna S. Roberts. *The Commonsense Guide to Weight Loss for People with Diabetes.* Alexandria, Va.: American Diabetes Association, 1998.

Highhopesfund.net. "NEJM Study Shows Fiber's Great Benefits in Type 2 Diabetes." Joslin Diabetes Center. 14 Mar. 2001 <www.highhopesfund.net/news/fiber_benefits.html>.

Hiser, Elizabeth. *The Other Diabetes.* New York: William Morrow and Company, 1999.

Hoogwerf, Byron, and Hertzel C. Gerstein. "The HOPE Study." *Practical Diabetology* Sept. 2000: 19–26.

"How Much Do You Know about Using Herbal Therapies?" *Diabetes Self-Management* Mar.-Apr. 2001: 48–49.

Hu, Frank B., et al. "Walking Compared with Vigorous Physical Activity and Risk of Type 2 Diabetes in Women." *Journal of the American Medical Association* 282, 15 (1999): 1433–39.

Huerta, R., et al. "Symptoms at the Menopausal and Pre-Menopausal Years: Their Relationship with Insulin, Glucose, Cortisol, FSH, Prolactin, Obesity and Attitudes Towards Sexuality." *Psychoneuroendocrinology* 20, 8 (1995): 851–64.

jdf.org. "Diabetes & Nerve Disease." Juvenile Diabetes Foundation International, April 1998. www.jdf.org/jdfliving

Joshi, Nirmal, et al. "Infections in Patients with Diabetes Mellitus." *The New England Journal of Medicine* 341, 25 (1999): 1906–12.

joslin.org. "Preventing Heart Disease, Stroke, Poor Circulation." Joslin Diabetes Center, Managing Diabetes, 2001. http://www.joslin.org/educa-tion/library/preventing.html.

Kahn, Ronald C., and Gordon C. Weir, eds. *Joslin's Diabetes Mellitus.* 13th ed. Baltimore: Williams and Wilkins, 1994.

Kaye, S. A., A. R. Folsom, J. M. Sprafka, F. J. Prineas, and R. B. Wallace. "Increased Incidence of Diabetes Mellitus in Relation to Abdominal Adiposity in Older Women." *Clinical Epidemiology* 44(3):329–34 (1991).

kidney.org. "Ten Facts About Diabetes and Kidney Disease." National Kidney Foundation, March 2001. http://www.kidney.org/general/news/diabetes.cfm.

Klag, Michael J., editor in chief, et al. *Johns Hopkins Family Health Book.* New York: HarperCollins Publishers, 1999.

Kruger, Davida F. *The Diabetes Travel Guide.* Alexandria, Va.: American Dia-betes Association, Inc., 2000.

Kurtzweil, Paula. "The New Food Label: Coping with Diabetes." Online post-ing. Nov. 1994, updated Sept. 1995. Food and Drug Administration. 16 Nov. 2000 http://www.vm.csfan.fda.gov/~dms/fdacdial.html.

Leontos, Carolyn. *What to Eat When You Get Diabetes.* New York: John Wiley and Sons, Inc., 2000.

Levin, Marvin E., and Michael A. Pfeifer, eds. *The Uncomplicated Guide to Diabetes Complications.* Alexandria, Va.: American Diabetes Association, Inc., 1998.

Liebman, Bonnie. "Exercise: Use It or Lose It!" *Nutrition Action* 22, 10 (1995): 1–7.

Lopez-Lopez, R., R. Huerta, and J. M. Malacar. "Age at Menopause in Women with Type 2 Diabetes Mellitus." *Menopause,* Summer 1999, 6(2):174–8.

Lorenz, Rodney A., et al. "Changing Behavior: Practical Lessons from the Di-abetes Control and Complications Trial." *Diabetes Care* 19, 6 (1996): 648–52.

Malacar, J. M., R. Huerta, B. Ribera, S. Esparza, and M. E. Fajardo. "Menopause in Normal and Uncomplicated NIDDM Women; Physical and Emotional Symptoms and Hormone Profile." *Maturitis.* Sept. 1997, 28(1):35–45.

Manson, JoAnn E., et al. "A Prospective Study of Exercise and Incidence of Diabetes among U.S. Male Physicians." *Journal of the American Medical Association* 268, 1 (1992): 63–64.

———. "Physical Activity and Incidence of Non-Insulin-Dependent Dia-betes Mellitus in Women." *The Lancet* 338 (1991): 774–78.

Marshall, J. A., et al. "High-Fat, Low-Carbohydrate Diet and the Etiology of

Non-Insulin-Dependent Diabetes Mellitus: The San Luis Valley Diabetes Study." *American Journal of Epidemiology* 134, 6 (1991): 590–603.

Mayer-Davis, Elizabeth J., et al. "Intensity and Amount of Physical Activity in Relation to Insulin Sensitivity." *Journal of the American Medical Association* 279, 9 (1998) 669–74.

McGarry, J. Denis. "Glucose-Fatty Acid Interactions in Health and Disease." *American Journal of Clinical Nutrition* 67 (suppl) (1998): 500S–4S.

Mitchell, Emma. *Energy Now: Simple Ways to Gain Vitality, Overcome Tension, and Achieve Harmony and Balance*. New York: Macmillan USA, 1998.

Motamedi, Beatrice. "African-Americans: A High Risk Group." Diabetes. com, April 2000.

nidcr.nih.gov. "Diabetes and Periodontal Disease: A Guide for Patients." National Institute of Dental and Craniofacial Research Publications Page. www.nidcr.nih.gov/news/pubs/diabetes/main.htm

niddk.nih.gov. "Alternative Therapies to Diabetes." National Diabetes Information Clearinghouse. 19 Jan. 2001. http://www.niddk.nih.gov/health/diabetes/summary/altmed/altmed. htm

niddk.nih.gov. "Diabetes in Hispanic Americans." National Diabetes Information Clearinghouse, 2000. www.niddk.nih.gov/health/diabetes/pubs/hispan/hispan.htm

niddk.nih.gov. "Kidney Disease of Diabetes." National Diabetes Information Clearinghouse. NIH Publication No. 01–3925, July 1995, updated April 2001. www.niddk.nih.gov/health/kidney/pubs/kdd/kdd.htm

niddk.nih.gov. "Medicines for People with Diabetes." National Diabetes Information Clearinghouse. 15 Nov. 2000. http://niddk.nih.gov/health/diabetes/pubs/med/index.htm

niddk.nih.gov. "Take Care of Your Feet for a Lifetime: A Guide for People with Diabetes." NIH Publication No. 01-4285, November 1997. http://ndep.nih.gov/materials/pubs/feet/brochure/index.htm

"Nutrition Recommendations and Principles for People with Diabetes Mellitus." *Diabetes Care* 20 (1997): S14–17.

Pasquariello, Patrick, Jr., M.D., Senior Editor. *The Children's Hospital of Philadelphia Book of Pregnancy and Child Care*. New York: John Wiley & Sons, 1999.

Pastors, Joyce Green, et al. "Psyllium Fiber Reduces Rise in Postprandial Glucose and Insulin Concentrations in Patients with Non-Insulin-Dependent Diabetes." *American Journal of Clinical Nutrition* 53 (1991): 1431–35.

Pinhas-Hamiel, O., et al. "The Type 2 Family: A Setting for the Development and Treatment of Adolescent Type 2 Diabetes Mellitus." *Archives of Pediatric Adolescent Medicine* 153, 10 (1999): 1063–67.

Poirer, Laurinda M., and Katharine M. Coburn. *Women & Diabetes: Life Planning for Health and Wellness*. 2nd ed. Alexandria, Va.: American Diabetes Association, 2000.

————. *Women & Diabetes: Life Planning for Health and Wellness*. Alexandria, Va.: American Diabetes Association, 1997.

"Resource Guide 2001." *Diabetes Forecast* 54, 1 (2001): 33–50.

Ritz, Eberhard, and Stephan Reinhold Orth. "Nephropathy in Patients with Type 2 Diabetes Mellitus." *The New England Journal of Medicine* 341, 15 (1999): 1127–33.

The Role of Frequent Glucose Monitoring in Intensive Diabetes Management. New York: The Resource Group, 2000.

Rosenthal, M. Sara. *The Type 2 Diabetic Woman*. Los Angeles: Lowell House, 1999.

Ross, Carolyn, et al. "Given Diabetes, Is Fat Better than Thin?" *Diabetes Care* 20, 4 (1997): 650–52.

Ruderman, N., A. Z. Apelian, and S. H. Schneider. "Exercise in Therapy and Prevention of Type II Diabetes. Implications for Blacks." *Diabetes Care* 13, 11 (1990): 1163–68.

Ruderman, Neil, and John T. Devlin, eds. *The Health Professional's Guide to Diabetes and Exercise*. Alexandria, Va.: American Diabetes Association, Inc., 1995.

Salmeron, Jorge, et al. "Dietary Fiber, Glycemic Load, and Risk of NIDDM in Men." *Diabetes Care* 20, 4 (1997): 545–50.

Sapolsky, Robert M. *Why Zebras Don't Get Ulcers: An Updated Guide to Stress, Stress-Related Diseases, and Coping*. New York: W. H. Freeman and Company, 2000.

Sizer, Frances, and Eleanor Whitney. *Nutrition: Concepts and Controversies*. 8th ed. Belmont, Calif., Wadsworth/Thomas Learning, 2000.

Streja, Daniel. "Blood Glucose Meters with Storage Capability." *Practical Diabetology* Sept. 2000: 7–18.

Surwit, Richard S., and Mark N. Feinglos. "The Effects of Relaxation on Glucose Tolerance in Non-Insulin-Dependent Diabetes." *Diabetes Care* 6, 2 (1983): 176–79.

Tamada, Janet A., et al. "Noninvasive Glucose Monitoring." *Journal of the American Medical Association* 282, 19 (1999): 1839–44.

Testa, Marcia A., and Donald C. Simonson. "Health Economic Benefits and Quality of Life During Improved Glycemic Control in Patients with Type 2 Diabetes Mellitus." *Journal of the American Medical Association* 380, 17 (1998): 1490–96.

Thomas, Maria. *The Unofficial Guide to Living with Diabetes*. New York: Macmillan, 1999.

Tuomilehto, Jaakko, et al. "Prevention of Type 2 Diabetes Mellitus by Changes in Lifestyle among Subjects with Impaired Glucose Tolerance." *The New England Journal of Medicine* 344, 18 (2001): 1343–50.

Turner, Robert C., et al. "Glycemic Control with Diet, Sulfonylurea, Metformin, or Insulin in Patients with Type 2 Diabetes Mellitus." *Journal of the American Medical Association* 281, 21 (1999): 2005–12

Valmadrid, Charles T., et al. "Alcohol Intake and the Risk of Coronary Heart Disease Mortality in Persons with Older-Onset Diabetes Mellitus." *Journal of the American Medical Association* 282, 3 (1999): 239–46.

Van Der Does, Ferdinand E. E., et al. "Symptoms and Well-Being in Relation to Glycemic Control in Type II Diabetes." *Diabetes Care* 19, 3 (1996): 204–8.

Wannamethee, S. G., et al. "Hypertension, Serum Insulin, Obesity and the Metabolic Syndrome." *Journal of Human Hypertension* 12, 11 (1998): 735–41.

Warshaw, Hope S. *Diabetes Meal Planning Made Easy.* 2nd ed. Alexandria, Va.: American Diabetes Association, Inc., 2000.

Warshaw, Hope S., and Karen M. Bolderman. *Practical Carbohydrate Counting.* Alexandria, Va.: American Diabetes Association, Inc., 2001.

Wei, Ming, et al. "Low Cardiorespiratory Fitness and Physical Inactivity as Predictors of Mortality in Men with Type 2 Diabetes." *Annals of Internal Medicine* 132, 8 (2000): 605–11.

Weil, Andrew. *8 Weeks to Optimum Health.* New York: Ballantine, 1997.

Weintraub, Michael I. "Chronic Submaximal Magnetic Stimulation in Peripheral Neuropathy: Is There a Beneficial Therapeutic Relationship?" *American Journal of Pain Management* 8, 1 (1998): 12–16.

"What to Know . . . Head to Toe." *Diabetes Forecast* May 2001: 107.

United States Department of Agriculture/Human Nutrition Information Service. *The Food Guide Pyramid.* Home and Garden Bulletin No. 252. Washington, D.C.: GPO, 1992.

United States Department of Health and Human Services, and National Institute of Diabetes and Digestive Kidney Diseases. *Feet Can Last a Lifetime.* Washington, D.C.: GPO, 1997.

United States Department of Health and Human Services, National Institutes of Health, and National Diabetes Information Clearinghouse. *Diabetes in African Americans.* NIH Publication No. 98-3266. Washington, D.C.: GPO, 1998.

Index